# The Official CNA Study Guide

CERTIFIED NURSING ASSISTANT PRACTICE TEST
AND SKILLS TEST FOR THE NNAAP EXAM

## Deborah Clark

Aegis Group LLC

The Complete CNA Study Guide
Copyright © 2015 by Aegis Group LLC

**Disclaimer**
Every effort has been made to ensure that the content provided on this book is accurate and helpful for our readers at publishing time. However, this is not an exhaustive treatment of the subjects and as you probably know, different States have different requirements and readings. No liability is assumed for losses or damages due to the information provided. You are responsible for your own choices, actions, and results.

*To all of the incredible Certified Nursing Assistants out there taking care of the sick and needy. Your job does not receive enough praise for the incredible and meaningful work you do time in and time out.*

*This book is dedicated to previous, current and soon to be CNAs everywhere.*

# Contents

# INTRODUCTION

The nursing profession is one of the most important professions in the health care field. This is because nurses are at the forefront of patient care, performing myriad functions all in the aim to assist their patients into healing, recovery, and whenever possible, an improved state of health. Some individuals in the nursing community are the CNAs. CNAs, or Certified Nursing Assistants, are significant members of the nursing profession since they are on the forefront and lend their valuable assistance to other members of the nursing profession in caring for patients.

CNAs do important tasks that are vital to the health care profession such as taking patients' vital signs, assisting in putting them in the best possible or most comfortable position, and assisting with feeding.

These tasks require that CNAs be competent and possess the necessary skills to be able to care for their patients safely and effectively. To prove this competency, Certified Nursing Assistants must pass the competency exam.

## THE CNA COMPETENCY EXAM

For those who aspire to work as a CNA, an examination is a requirement prior to holding a valid CNA license, which is one of the most important requirements for practice. If you want to become a qualified CNA, the first thing you need to complete is a training course that involves both theoretical and practical knowledge on the job functions of a CNA. Training courses usually last 12 weeks on average and incorporate the concepts that are part of the examination. The CNA examination will also determine if you, as a practitioner, can work in different patient care settings such as hospitals or other care facilities like nursing homes.

The CNA exam is usually issued by the state in which you wish to practice, and therefore may vary in content depending on the state where you are taking it. Regardless of the variations however, the core concepts of the examinations are similar and there are two parts of the examinations given within the United States.

The most popular concepts covered in both the written and practical components of the exam are about your knowledge of different techniques in providing safe and effective patient care, principles of effective communication with the patient and other members of the health care team, and knowledge about safety guidelines and procedures. Successfully passing both the written and practical portions of the test allows you to work as a CNA in your respective state.

## Written Part of the Exam

The first part of the CNA examination is the written test. This is composed of multiple choice questions where you'll be asked to choose the best answer based on the situation provided in the question. Questions that are usually part of the written exam consist of concepts concerning nutrition and patient hygiene, control of infection, knowledge of different therapeutic procedures and practices, and maintenance of an appropriate conduct in the workplace. Also, part of the concept being tested in this part of the exam is how you are able to meet the psychosocial needs of your patients and their families, and your knowledge of different ethical considerations in caring for patients.

## Clinical Skills Test

The clinical skills section of the CNA exam tests your skills on actual provision of care for patients. This part will have you demonstrate different nursing tasks and activities on a model patient as the examiners assess and grade you on your skills. The most common skills you will be assessed for include obtaining blood pressure readings, feeding and bathing a patient, assisting in dressing an individual and the use of different equipment to carry out activities of daily living, such as bed pans and bedside commodes.

Furthermore, the practical component of the exam may also require an examinee to demonstrate assistance for a patient as he or she performs range of motion exercises and ambulation. Hand washing may also be part of those skills that would be tested as well as how a CNA observes proper communication and interaction with patients.

## Certification Standards

Becoming a certified nursing assistant is somewhat of a complex evolution. Unlike most certifications, CNA certification requirements are different for each state. Without a national standard, being certified in one state does not necessarily mean your certification will carry over to another state.

However, the difference between the Written Exams (WE) and the Critical Skills Exams (CSE) between different states is minimal. Furthermore, there is a standardized testing process that does allow you to transfer your certification between certain states.

The National Nurse Aide Assessment Program (NNAAP) is the largest nurse aide certification examination program in the United States with over 200,000 written and practical exams administered annually. Under the jurisdiction of the National Council of State Boards of Nursing (NCSBN), 25 states are now utilizing the NNAAP exam to measure the nurse aide basic level competency, namely:

Alabama, Alaska, California, Colorado, District of Columbia, Georgia, Guam, Louisiana, Mariana Islands, Maryland, Minnesota, Mississippi, New Hampshire, North Carolina, North Dakota, Pennsylvania, Rhode Island, South Carolina, Texas, Vermont, Virginia, Virgin Islands, Washington, Wisconsin, Wyoming

The development of the NNAAP test plan reflects the knowledge, abilities, and skills essential for the CNA candidate to meet patients' needs regarding health promotion, maintenance, and restoration of health. NNAAP test plan provisions are grounded on evidence-based practice of newly-certified nurse aides. These include CNA activities in relation to the significance of their performance, their impact on client safety, and the settings of care rendered.

So as to help best prepare you for the certification process, this study guide will use the structure and process of the NNAAP for the following reasons:

1. You have about a 50/50 chance of one day taking an NNAAP certification at some point in your career. Therefore, it is the most useful and pertinent of the certification processes to follow.

2. In order to convince states to relinquish control of their own certification process and adopt the NNAAP as a set standard, the NCSBN had to prove to each state that their certification process was a better indicator of qualification and presented a higher standard than what previously existed. Therefore, it can be assumed that the NNAAP is a more difficult process and requires more effort than other state exams.

3. Considering that 4 states have recently switched to the NNAAP, it can be understood that the number of states accepting NNAAP certification will only grow over the years. Being the leading standardized CNA certification process in the U.S., there is a chance it might one day be adopted by all the remaining states.

4. The NNAAP adheres to testing the CNA required competencies based on the quality assurance standard adhering to the OBRA guidelines, the federal regulation guidelines for nursing assistants/nurse aides.

The NNAAP has two components: a written or oral exam and a skills demonstration exam. A CNA candidate is required to complete both to qualify for the certification in a state and be added to the state nurse aide registry. The state registry is an assurance for employers that the CNA job applicant has met the necessary federal and state employment requirements.

## Certification Layout

### A. Written Examination

The written portion is comprised of 70 multiple-choice items, 10 of which are non-scored or pretest items for collection of statistical information.

The oral examination includes 60 multiple-choice items and 10 reading comprehension or word recognition items. The examinee may choose to take either the written or the oral examination.

The examination comprises three major domains: physical care skills, psychosocial care skills, and Role of the Nurse Aide. The sub domains are organized as follows:

| Content Domain | Weight | Number of items |
|---|---|---|
| **1. Physical Care Skills** | 60% | 36 |
|   A. Activities of Daily Living | 14% | 8 |
|   B. Basic Nursing Skills | 39% | 24 |
|   C. Restorative Skills | 7 % | 4 |
| **2. Psychosocial Care Skills** | 13% | 8 |
|   A. Emotional and Mental Health Needs | 11% | 6 |
|   B. Spiritual and Cultural Needs | 2% | 2 |
| **3. Role of the Nurse Aide** | 27% | 16 |
|   A. Communication | 8% | 5 |
|   B. Client Rights | 7% | 4 |
|   C. Legal and Ethical Behavior | 3% | 2 |
|   D. Member of the Health Care Team | 9% | 5 |
| Total | 100% | 60 |

**B. Clinical Skills Test**

In this second part of the examination, the candidate is required to demonstrate his/her competencies by performing five hands-on skills. These skills are randomly selected from a list of 25 CNA skills. A designated evaluator will grade each candidate on the performance of the selected nurse aide skills, which must be correctly completed within a given time frame in order to pass this exam.

The clinical skills test will be conducted in a setting simulating a nursing aide's working environment. All the necessary tools and equipment in the performance of the skills are made available. Before the start of the exam, the candidate is allowed to ask questions or raise points of clarifications. Twenty-five to thirty minutes are usually allocated for the performance of all five selected skills.

The 25 basic nurse aide skills from which the five skills shall be chosen for this exam include:

- Hand washing
- Apply one knee-high elastic stocking or anti-embolic stocking
- Assist to ambulate a client using transfer belt
- Assist client with use of bedpan
- Clean upper and lower dentures
- Count and record client's radial pulse
- Count and record patient's respirations
- Don and remove gown and gloves (PPE)
- Dress client with affected (weak) right arm
- Feed client who cannot feed self
- Give modified bed bath
- Make an occupied bed
- Measure and record blood pressure
- Measure and record urinary output
- Measure and record weight of ambulatory client
- Perform passive range of motion exercises for client knee and ankle
- Perform passive range of motion exercises for client shoulder
- Position client on side
- Provide catheter care for female client
- Provide fingernail care
- Provide food care
- Provide mouth care
- Provide perineal care for female client
- Transfer from bed to wheelchair using transfer belt
- Moving patient from bed to the stretcher

## Study Guide Layout

Judicious use of this study guide, either alone or with major nurse aide theoretical references, will help you achieve your goal of becoming a CNA. The Official CNA Study Guide gives you the essentials you need to pass the examination. Guidelines, test taking tips, test-based focus concepts and sample questions are provided to prepare you for the actual types of questions you'll see during the scheduled exam.

To begin your CNA certification preparations, we will begin by administering a pretest. The idea behind the pretest is to help decipher what areas of the CNA examination you need the most help with. If you find that you did worse in a particular section over the others, then it is our recommendation that you spend more time preparing in that particular section.

Once you have completed the pretest and understand your scoring, you can move on to the study guide.

The study guide portion consists of 9 chapters based on the 9 NNAAP categories. Each chapter follows a well-designed structure with cues and highlights to aid you in mastering the concepts and developing your critical analysis and test-taking skills. The concepts are patterned from the NNAAP exam blueprint by the NCSBN covering the different domains being measured in the certification examination.

Each chapter begins with a list of terms to learn and understand, followed by the details of the "must-knows." Commonly asked concepts in the actual exam are also highlighted in every section.

The coverage of the main categories and thus the different chapter titles are:

- Activities of Daily Living
- Basic Nursing Skills
- Restorative Skills
- Emotional and Mental Health Needs
- Spiritual and Cultural Needs
- Communication
- Clients Rights
- Legal and Ethical Behavior
- Member of the Health Care Team

Finally, so as to help you with your own assessment, we will provide two sets of integrated practice exams. The questions are constructed to gauge your strengths and weaknesses and to develop the necessary skills in attacking actual test items.Let's begin.

# PRETEST

One of the best and most effective learning plans is one that starts with a self-assessment of your current status. You need to understand what kind of learner you are, the learning strategies that suit you best, the coverage of the examination and your areas of strengths and weaknesses.

To best prepare you for this, we have devised a Pretest. The results of the pretest enable you to create a more organized and effective review plan in terms of effectively allocating your time, effort, and resources in the different areas of the test framework.

This pretest consists of 25 integrated multiple-choice questions from the nine key areas of the actual exam. Item analysis is done at the end this test to determine your performance in the different categories. A brief discussion of the correct answers is also available in this section.

Once you are finished with the exam, score up your points and keep special attention to the "AREA" category at the end. Tally up the results and see which category you had the lowest score in.

Keep in mind that the results of this test are not indicative of whether or not you are ready for the final exam.

# PRETEST QUESTIONS

1. The nurse aide is preparing to transfer a patient to another unit. To increase stability during client transfer, the nurse aide increases the base of support by performing which of the following?

    A. Leaning slightly backward

    B. Spacing the feet further apart

    C. Tensing the abdominal muscles

    D. Bending the knees

2. A nurse aide is caring for a client weighing 250 pounds. Which of the following reflects the nurse aide's awareness of workplace injury?

    A. Using proper body mechanics will prevent injuries

    B. As long as he is physically fit, there is lesser risk of injury when transferring the client

    C. He uses mechanical lift and asks another person's assistance to transfer the client from the bed to the chair

    D. He uses the back belt to avoid straining his back

3. While making the bed of the client, the nurse aide finds a needle on the bed sheet. What should the nurse aide do with it?

    A. Pick it carefully and place it on the client's bedside table

    B. Place it in the client's medication storage

    C. Dispose it the client's trash bin

    D. Dispose it in the sharps or puncture-resistant container

4. The nurse aide is changing the client's bed linens. Which of the following techniques is inappropriate in performing the activity?

    A. She folds the contaminated side of the linen inwards

    B. She places the contaminated linens in a plastic bag

    C. She drops the linens on the floor while changing them

D. She changes the contaminated linens as soon as noticing them

5. When caring for a cerebrovascular accident (CVA) client with right-sided weakness, what part of the upper garment is put on first?

A. Right sleeve

B. Left sleeve

C. Both sleeves

D. Client's preference

6. Ideally, for **therapeutic communication** to be effective the members of the team must be aware of how they communicate with the client. Which of the following is not classified as a verbal communication?

A. Clarifying the client's statements

B. Asking the client open-ended questions

C. Using leading questions to encourage client to verbalize

D. Use of eye contact and gestures

7. The main purpose of padding and keeping the bedside rails up is to:

A. Serve as an attachment area to secure the call bell

B. Keep the client safely restrained on bed

C. Serve as a support for the client to reposition himself on bed

D. Promote safety and prevent injuries to the client

8. While assisting a client with denture care the nurse aide observes that the upper plate is cracked. The nurse aide's most appropriate action at this time is to:

A. Notify the nurse-in-charge of the damage

B. Assist the client in making an appointment with the dentist in his convenient time

C. Clean the dentures thoroughly before returning to the client's mouth

D. Soak the denture in an oral aseptic, rinse, dry thoroughly then use adhesives to address the crack

9. Depending on the health of the client's mouth, special care may be needed every 2 to 8 hours. To prevent liquid from draining down the client's throat, the client should be:

   A.  Assisted to sitting position in bed, if health permits, or if not, to side-lying position with head turned

   B.  Assisted to lying position, if health permits, or if not, transferred to a chair

   C.  Placed in a sitting position at the edge of the bed leaning over a bedside table

   D.  Placed in any position of comfort

10. Gloves should be worn as personal protective equipment when performing which of the following activities?

   A.  Taking the vital signs of a client

   B.  Handing the bedpan of the client

   C.  Feeding the client with regular meals

   D.  Assisting the client in ambulation

11. The CNA is attending to the care of a 75-year-old bedridden female client. While performing backrub, she noticed changes in the skin integrity of the elderly. Which one indicates the beginning of a pressure sore?

   A.  Swelling

   B.  Pain

   C.  Numbness

   D.  Discoloration

12. The nurse aide enters the room of a middle-aged male client, and he claims that he has severe pain. What is the best action of the nurse aide?

   A.  Acknowledge the client's statements and proceed to usual activities

   B.  Tell the client to ambulate for a while to alleviate the pain

   C.  Report the client's concern to the nurse-in-charge

D. Assure the client that the pain will go away soon

13. In dealing with client's care, the nurse aide keeps in mind that the client has the right to:

   A. Access other client's chart in the area

   B. Smoke and roam around in the facility

   C. Entertain visitors anytime

   D. Have access to mail and telephone

14. A client has been very talkative and unruly, so the nurse aide isolated him in the closet for an hour. The nurse aide is liable for:

   A. False imprisonment

   B. Neglect

   C. Battery

   D. Involuntary seclusion

15. The nurse aide is pulled out and transferred to another unit requiring additional manpower. She accepts a new assignment without complaint. She is demonstrating what personal working trait?

   A. Accountability

   B. Flexibility

   C. Being considerate

   D. Self-autonomy

16. Members of the health care team are required to observe the use of isolation procedures based on the client's condition. Which statement best reflects the purpose of using isolation protocols?

   A. To ensure client's privacy

   B. To organize functional bedside care tasks

   C. To control or minimize the spread of infection

   D. To save time and effort of the team

17. In reporting unusual occurrences in the care of client or certain incidents, the nurse aide understands that:

    A. Only accidents or incidents related to malpractice require an incident report to be completed

    B. All accidents and incidents require an incident report to be completed

    C. Only accidents or incidents that result in injury require an incident report to be completed

    D. Only the person involved or injured is required to complete an incident report

18. All but one of these nurse aide activities can promote sleep for the clients:

    A. Provide emotional support when client experiences pain

    B. Assist the client with the use of positioning devices to enhance comfort

    C. Decrease noise and confusion in the client's environment

    D. Change the client's routine regularly to provide diversion

19. One of your responsibilities in the care of a dependent client who cannot move or ambulate on his own is performing passive range of motion (PROM) exercises. Which of the following statements is not an advantage of PROM?

    A. Prevents muscle atrophy

    B. Improves client's nutrition

    C. Promotes circulation

    D. Increases joint movements

20. In attending to an immobilized client, the nurse aide knows that he is at risk of the following complications of immobility, EXCEPT:

    A. Pneumonia

    B. Increased nutritional intake

    C. Bed sores

    D. Muscle atrophy

21. A nurse aide who is active in a religious congregation is assigned to a client of different religious background. The nurse aide should:

A. Emphasize the importance of joining a religious group or church to the client even if it's of a different sect

B. Respect the client's beliefs and refrain from starting religious discussions

C. Ask the clergyman from their church to visit the client

D. Make the client understand the nurse aide's faith

22. A terminally ill client says, "Why me? God is punishing me!" The nurse aide best responds by:

A. Acknowledging the client's feelings and listening quietly

B. Make jokes to divert the client

C. Say, "God doesn't punish people with illness."

D. Ignore the client's statements

23. How does a nurse aide appropriately assist a client with his spiritual needs?

A. Encouraging the client to talk about his beliefs

B. Avoiding any religious discussions to prevent arguments

C. Talking about the nurse aide's own religious beliefs

D. Bringing the client to the nurse aide's religious group for indoctrination

24. After providing morning care, the client offers the nurse aide a fifty dollar bill as an appreciation for her service. Which action is most appropriate for the nurse aide to do?

A. Accept the money to avoid offending the client

B. Politely refuse the client's offer

C. Contact the nurse-in-charge what to do

D. Accept the money and buy food for the entire team

25. Which of the following facilitates effective communication with a client suffering from total hearing loss?

    A.   Smile and talk slowly

    B.   Smile often and talk loudly

    C.   Write out information and instructions for the client to read

    D.   Allow the client more time to talk

# PRETEST ANSWERS AND RATIONALE

1. ANSWER: B. Spacing the feet further apart

    RATIONALE: The key word in this question is "base," and the feet will provide for this foundation of stability. Leaning backward will cause back strain and decrease balance.

    AREA: Basic Nursing Skills

2. ANSWER: C. He uses a mechanical lift and asks another person's assistance to transfer the client from the bed to the chair

    RATIONALE: It is prudent to always keep in mind the proper use of body mechanics to decrease risk of injuries, while understanding the importance of using assistive devices and employing the help of other staff as needed.

    AREA: Basic Nursing Skills

3. ANSWER: D. Dispose it in the sharps or puncture-resistant container

    RATIONALE: Sharps and needles without being recapped should be disposed in sharps container or puncture-resistant container to prevent accidental pricks and possible transmission of blood borne pathogens.

    AREA: Basic Nursing Skills

4. ANSWER: C. She dropped the linens on the floor while changing them

    RATIONALE: Dropping linens on the floor will lead to contamination and promotes spread of micro-organisms.

    AREA: Basic Nursing Skills

5. ANSWER: A. Right sleeve

    RATIONALE: Affected side should be dressed first to avoid further shearing of garments on the area.

    AREA: Activities of Daily Living

6. ANSWER: D. Use of eye contact and gestures

RATIONALE: Nonverbal communication is the process of communication through sending and receiving wordless cues. It includes the use of gestures, posture, facial expressions, eye contact and physical distance.

AREA: Communication

7. ANSWER: D. Promote safety and prevent injuries to the client

RATIONALE: Padding the side rails and keeping them up prevents injuries like falls and direct physical trauma. The side rails should not be used as an attachment frame for call bells, tubes, and other devices.

AREA: Basic Nursing Skills

8. ANSWER: A. Notify the nurse-in-charge of the damage

RATIONALE: Cracked and ill-fitting dentures can cause oral injuries and should not be continuously worn by the client. The nurse-in-charge should be notified for alternative oral interventions and collaboration with the dental team.

AREA: Basic Nursing Skills

9. ANSWER: A. Assisted to sitting position in bed

RATIONALE: Keeping the client in an upright position, if not contraindicated, or on the side prevents aspiration of secretions and oral hygiene fluids.

AREA: Activities of Daily Living

10. ANSWER: B. Handling the bedpan of the client

RATIONALE: Potential exposure to client's body secretions and waste like urine and excreta requires the use of gloves as part of the contactor enteric precautions to prevent contamination and further spread of pathogens. Taking vital signs, feeding, and ambulating the client do not necessitate the use of gloves.

AREA: Activities of Daily Living

11. ANSWER: D. Discoloration

RATIONALE: Stage I or the earliest stage of a pressure ulcer is non-blanchable reddish discoloration of the skin. Prolonged bed rest and pressure on dependent areas of the body results in compromised circulation in the underlying affected areas, leading to skin breakdown.

AREA: Basic Nursing Skills

12. ANSWER: C. Report the client's concern to the nurse-in-charge

RATIONALE: The client's pain needs to be further assessed by the nurse-in-charge to determine the necessary interventions to be done. Client's complaint of pain should be acknowledged and addressed before proceeding to other activities.

AREA: Member of the Health Care Team

13. ANSWER: D. Have access to mail and telephone

RATIONALE: Patient rights are those basic rules of conduct between patients and medical caregivers as well as the institutions and people that support them. Examples of patient rights include the right to information and communication (telephones, emails, information regarding his care), the right to quality care and treatment, the right to refuse treatment, and the right to informed consent.

AREA: Clients Rights

14. ANSWER: D. Involuntary seclusion

RATIONALE: Involuntary seclusion is the act of punishing a client by isolating him or her from others. In this case, the client was isolated in a closet as a form of punishment. False imprisonment is when a client is restrained from moving freely about against his or her will. Invasion of privacy occurs when the nurse aide fails to keep the client's information confidential. Neglect is an act resulting to harm or injury due to the non-performance of an expected action to meet client's needs.

AREA: Legal and Ethical Behaviors

15. ANSWER: B. Flexibility

RATIONALE: Flexibility is a trait in which a nurse aide would accept a new assignment without complaint. A nurse aide would most likely be re-assigned to a new area or unit and flexibility is needed to deal with the disruption in work routine. Being considerate is being thoughtful, kind, and caring toward others. Self-autonomy is acting responsibly on the right decisions and performance of necessary activities including self-management. Accountability is performing duties with responsibility to the outcomes of such actions.

AREA: Member of the Health Care Team

16. ANSWER: C. To control or minimize the spread of infection

RATIONALE: Isolation protocols for the use of personal protective equipment (PPE) described by the Center for Disease Control and being implemented by health care facilities are designed to control, prevent, or minimize the spread of infection. These include the different precautions such as standard, contact, airborne, and respiratory isolations with the use of principles in asepsis.

AREA: Basic Nursing Skills

17. ANSWER: B. All accidents and incidents require an incident report to be completed

RATIONALE: All accidents and incidents require an incident report to be completed regardless of whether the incident resulted in actual injuries or not. All members of the team involved, including witnesses, are required to complete an incident report. Facilities use incident reports to improve their quality of health care delivery services.

AREA: Legal and Ethical Behavior

18. ANSWER: D. Change the client's routine regularly to provide diversion

RATIONALE: Changing the client's routine regularly would disrupt his/her habits and may cause confusion and agitation causing impaired sleep patterns. Regular and highly structured routines can better promote comfort and decrease the client's anxiety.

AREA: Activities of Daily Living

19. ANSWER: B. Improves client's nutrition

RATIONALE: PROM will not directly improve the client's appetite or increase nutritional intake but can help prevent muscle atrophy, contractures, and deformities. PROM can also help improve circulation, joint mobility, and client's mood.

AREA: Restorative Skills

20. ANSWER: B Increased nutritional intake

RATIONALE: Complications of immobility include pneumonia, atelectasis and respiratory infections due to stasis of lung secretions and decreased lung capacity. Circulation is also compromised resulting in bed sores, thrombus formation and muscle deformities. Immobilized clients usually cannot take adequate food on their own.

AREA: Restorative Skills

21. ANSWER: B. Respect the client's beliefs and refrain from starting religious discussions

THE OFFICIAL CNA STUDY GUIDE • 19

RATIONALE: Members of the team should acknowledge and respect the spiritual beliefs of the client and avoid imposing their own religion or cultural practices.

AREA: Spiritual and Cultural Needs

22. ANSWER: A. Acknowledging the client's feelings and listening quietly

RATIONALE: The client is experiencing expected grieving reactions under the anger stage. The nurse aide can be therapeutic by acknowledging the client's reactions and feelings in the grieving process without judgment and encouraging the client to verbalize or express his or her concerns.

AREA: Emotional and Mental Needs

23. ANSWER: A. Encouraging the client to talk about his beliefs

RATIONALE: Respecting and allowing the client to express his spiritual beliefs promotes well-being and fulfillment of the client's spiritual needs. Individualities and diversities in beliefs and religion should be respected without imposing one's own beliefs on the client.

AREA: Spiritual and Cultural Needs

24. ANSWER: B. Politely refuse the client's offer

RATIONALE: Accepting personal favors and tokens from the client is unprofessional and against work ethics. It is the responsibility of the health care team to render unconditional quality care to clients in the facility.

AREA: Legal and Ethical Behaviors

25. ANSWER: C. Write out information and instructions for the client to read

RATIONALE: Deaf clients can't hear verbal messages but benefit most in the use of nonverbal communication like the use of pen and paper, picture boards, or written instructions in the communication process.

AREA: Communication

# Scoring

Use the following table of specifications provided below for the pre-test in doing item analysis of each question to determine key areas of strengths and weaknesses in the 9 main categories of CNA exam.

**Table of pretest specifications:**

| Category | Percentage | Number of items |
|---|---|---|
| Activities of Daily Living | 16% | 4 |
| Basic Nursing Skills | 32% | 8 |
| Restorative Skills | 8% | 2 |
| Emotional and Mental Health Needs | 4% | 1 |
| Spiritual and Cultural Needs | 8% | 2 |
| Communication | 8% | 2 |
| Clients Rights | 4% | 1 |
| Legal and Ethical Behavior | 12% | 3 |
| Member of the Health Care Team | 8% | 2 |
| | 100% | 25 |

# ACTIVITIES OF DAILY LIVING

## TERMS TO REMEMBER:

- **Activities of Daily Living:** These are the basic tasks of everyday activity that a person would normally go through to include eating, bathing, dressing, etc.

- **Cleaning Bath:** A bath that was made for the sole purpose of helping a client get cleaned whether from daily activity or because they have soiled themselves.

- **Therapeutic Bath:** A bath that is given for medical purposes such as the removal or crust or dead skin, or the application of medication.

- **Tepid Bath:** Tepid is used to infer that it is a luke-warm bath for either cleaning or therapeutics means.

- **Sulcular Technique:** Teeth brushing technique that employs a circular motion around the bass of the bums and through the tooth. Also known as the bass technique.

- **Foot Hygiene:** Care to a patients foot to include cleaning and caring for.

- **Oral Hygiene:** Care to a patient's mouth through cleaning, brushing, flossing and denture care.

- **Hair Care:** Care of a patient's hair to include cleaning, brushing, etc…

Activities of Daily Living (ADLs), also referred to as "self-care skills" or "life skills," are everyday activities and functions an individual performs to live an independent, healthy life.

Basic ADLs are those that include dressing oneself, oral hygiene, making the bed, bathing, elimination activities, and eating.

Complex ADLs extend to household chores, child care, preparing meals, driving, social activities, and earning a living. Clients may experience struggle in performing ADLs due to health deficits at certain degrees like alterations in physiologic and psychosocial integrity.

Hence, it is part of the nurse aide's responsibilities to assist them in the performance of these routines to promote optimal health and function.

## BATHING

- Bathing removes accumulated oil, perspirations, dead skin cells, and some microorganisms.

- Stimulates circulation.

  - A warm or hot bath dilates superficial arterioles, bringing more blood and nourishment to the skin.

  - Rubbing with long smooth strokes from the distal to the proximal parts of extremities (from the point farthest from the body to the point closest) facilitates venous blood return.

- Produces sense of well-being.

**Categories of Baths.** There are two categories: cleaning and therapeutic baths.

1. CLEANING BATHS: Given for hygiene purposes.

   Temperature: 43°C to 46°C (110°F to115°F)

   a. Complete Bed Bath: The nurse aide washes the entire body of a dependent client on a bed.

   b. Self-Help Bath: Client is able to bathe himself with assistance from the nurse aide.

   c. Partial Bath (Abbreviated bath): Only specific neglected parts of the body are washed: the face, hands, axilla, perineal area and back.

   d. Bag Bath: This is a commercially prepared product with 10 to 12 presoaked disposable washcloths with no-rinse cleanser solution. The package is warmed in the microwave for 1 minute and used to clean each area of the body.

   e. Tub Baths: Tub baths are preferred over bed baths if permitted by a client's condition, because it is easier to wash and rinse the client.

   f. Shower: Ambulatory clients are able to use a shower in the facility with minimal assistance. In long-term facilities, a shower chair may be provided to aid in bathing.

2. THERAPEUTIC BATHS: These are given to promote physical effects, such as soothing irritated skin or to treat a specific area.

Temperature: The bath temperature is generally included in the order: 37.7°C to 46°C (100°F to 115°F) for adults, and 40.5°C (105°F) for infants.

- Medications may be added in the water bath.

- A therapeutic bath is generally taken in a tub one-third or one-half full.

- The client remains in the bath for 20 to 30 minutes.

## Pointers in Performing Baths:

- For clients receiving intravenous therapy, use easy-to-remove gowns that have Velcro or snap fasteners along the sleeves

- Provide client privacy by drawing the curtains or closing the door.

- Rationale: Hygiene is a personal matter.

- Position bed at comfortable working height. Lower the side rail on the side close to you. Assist client to move near you.

  Rationale: This prevents undue reaching and straining and promotes use of good body mechanics.

- Place a bath blanket over the top sheet then remove the top sheet from under the bath blanket by starting at the shoulders moving down toward the feet.

  Rationale: The bath blanket provides comfort, warmth, and privacy.

  Note: If the bed linen is to be reused, place it over the bedside chair. If it is to be changed, place it in the linen hamper, NEVER on the floor.

- Make a bath mitt with the washcloth.

  Rationale: A bath mitt retains water and heat better than a cloth loosely held and prevents ends of washcloth from dragging across the skin.

- In washing arms and hands, place a towel lengthwise under the arm away from you.

  Rationale: it protects soaking the bed.

- Use long, firm strokes from the wrist to the shoulder, including axillary area. For the legs and feet, from the ankle to the knee to the thigh.

Rationale: Firm strokes from distal to proximal areas promote circulation by increasing venous blood return.

- In washing the back, turn the client into a prone or side-lying position away from you. Wash from the shoulders to the buttocks and upper thighs.

## PERINEAL-GENITAL CARE

- ALERT: Always wash or wipe from "clean to dirty."

  - Female client: cleanse the perineal area from front to back.

  - Male client: cleanse the urinary meatus by moving in a circular motion from center of urethral opening around the penis.

- Nurse aides should wear gloves while providing this care for the client to protect themselves from infection.

*Pointers in Performing Perineal Care:*

Female Client:

- Place in back-lying position with knees flexed and spread well apart.

- Use separate quarters of washcloth for each stroke, and wipe from pubis to rectum.

  Rationale: Using separate quarters of the washcloth for new wipes prevents transmission of micro-organisms.

Male Client:

- Place in supine position with knees slightly flexed and hips slightly externally rotated.

- Wash and dry the penis using firm strokes.

- If uncircumcised, retract the prepuce or foreskin to expose the tip of the penis for cleaning.

  Rationale: Retracting the foreskin is necessary to remove the smegma, the thick cheesy secretion, that collects under the foreskin and facilitates bacterial growth.

## SKIN CARE

Dry Skin

- Use cleansing creams to clean the skin rather than soap or detergent, which causes drying, and in some, allergic reactions.

- Encourage client to drink more fluids.

- Use moisturizing or emollient creams that contain lanolin, petroleum jelly, or cocoa butter to maintain skin moisture.

Skin Rashes

- Wash the area with mild soap.

- Use tepid bath or soak to relieve itching. Caladryl lotion may also be indicated.

Acne

- Wash face with soap and warm water frequently to remove oil and dirt.

- Avoid oily creams and cosmetics that blocks the skin pores.

- Tell client to never squeeze or pick on the lesions.

## FOOT HYGIENE

Foot Problems

- Callus: thickened portion of the epidermis usually caused by pressure from shoes.

  - Soak foot in warm water with Epsom salts and abrade with pumice stones.

  - Apply lanolin cream.

- Corn: conical or circular keratosis caused by friction and pressure from the shoe and commonly occurs on the fourth or fifth toe.

  - Corns are generally addressed surgically.

  - Prevent recurrence by wearing comfortable shoes and massaging the area to promote circulation.

- Unpleasant odors: occur as a result of perspiration and its interaction with microbes.

  - Promote regular and frequent washing of the feet and wearing clean hosiery.

- Use foot powders and deodorants as needed.

- Plantar warts: appear on the soles of the foot and are caused by a virus. They are frequently painful and disrupt walking.

  - It is managed by the physician by curettage.

- Fissures: deep grooves often occur between toes as a result of dryness and cracking of the skin.

  - Provide good foot hygiene and application of an antiseptic to prevent infection.

- Athlete's foot: ringworm of the foot is caused by a fungus, characterized by scaling and cracking of the skin.

  - Treatment includes application of antifungal preparations.

  - Keep the feet well-ventilated, dry the feet well after bathing, and use clean socks.

- Ingrown toenail: an inward growth of the nail into soft tissues around it.

  - Preventing recurrence involves adherence to proper nail-trimming techniques.

## *Pointers in foot care:*

- File the nails straight across the ends of the toes.

- Encourage use of comfortable, well-fitting shoes.

- Avoid walking barefoot to prevent injury and infection.

- Avoid wearing constricting garments such as knee-high elastic stockings and avoid crossing legs which may impede foot circulation.

- Avoid self-treatment of corns and calluses.

- Fill washbasin with warm water at about 40°C to 43°C (105°F to110°F).

  Rationale: warm water promotes circulation, comfort, and is refreshing.

- Place pillow under the client's knees on bed.

  Rationale: This provides support and minimizes fatigue.

- If nails are brittle or thick and require trimming soak foot for 10 to 20 minutes.

Rationale: Soaking softens the nails and loosens debris under them.

## ORAL HYGIENE

- Note: Wear gloves when providing mouth care for partially or totally dependent clients to guard against infections.

Brushing the Teeth

- Assist the client to a sitting position in bed, if health permits. If not, assist the client to side-lying position with head turned.

    Rationale: To prevent fluid from draining down the throat.

- For client on bed, hold basin under the client's chin, fitting the small curve around the chin or neck.

- SULCULAR TECHNIQUE: Hold the toothbrush against the teeth with the bristles at a 45 degree angle with the tips of the outer bristles under the gum or gingival margins.

    Rationale: This technique removes plaque and cleans under the gum margins.

- Move the bristles up and down gently in short strokes from the sulcus or gums to the crown of the teeth.

- Brush tongue gently with toothbrush.

Flossing

    Note: Waxed floss is less likely to fray than unwaxed types.

- Wrap one end of the floss around the third finger of each hand.

- Use thumb and index finger to stretch the floss for the upper teeth.

- Gently slide the floss into the space between the gum and the tooth. Move the floss away from the gum with up and down motions.

Caring for Artificial Dentures

- Plate: complete set of artificial teeth for one jaw.

- Ill-fitting dentures, cracked dentures, or other defective oral prostheses can cause discomfort, injury, and chewing difficulties. Report any abnormalities in the dentures to the nurse-in-charge.

- Removing dentures:

    - Wear gloves. Use tissue or gauze, grasp the upper plate at the front teeth with the thumb and index fingers then move the denture up and down slightly.

        Rationale: The slight movement disrupts the suction that holds the plate on the roof of the mouth.

    - Lift the lower plate, turning it to the left side to remove the plate without stretching the lips.

- Cleaning dentures:

    - Take the denture container to a sink. Place a washcloth in the bowl of the sink to prevent damage if dentures are dropped.

    - Rinse dentures with tepid running water. Soak stained dentures in a denture cleaner.

## HAIR CARE

Hair Problems

- Dandruff: often accompanied by itching and appears as diffuse scaling of the scalp.

    - Usually treated effectively with shampoo.

- Hair loss: baldness could be related to aging, hereditary traits, or other underlying health conditions and treatment.

    - Encourage use of hairpiece, turban, or wig.

- Ticks: may include Rocky Mountain Spotted fever, Lyme disease and tularemia.

    - Use blunt tweezers to remove ticks. Gently pull the tick away using perpendicular motion.

- Lice: parasites that are easily transmitted through contact.

    - Treatment includes pediculosides such as pyrethrins, permethrin, and lindane.

    - Encourage use of fine-toothed nit combs and meticulous hair hygiene.

### *Pointers in Hair Care*

- Assist client who can sit to move to a chair or raise the head of the bed.

- Remove mats by pulling apart with fingers or with repeated brushings.

- Rub oil on the strands to help loosen very tangled hair.

- Comb out tangles in a small section of hair toward the ends. Stabilize the hair with one hand and comb toward the ends of the hair with the other hand.

  Rationale: This prevents scalp trauma.

- For short hair, brush or comb one side at a time. Divide long hair into two sections by parting it down the middle from the front to the back.

- Braiding long hairs prevents tangles.

## FEEDING THE CLIENT

- Assist in washing client's hands and providing mouth care as indicated.

- Position the bed in low position with the client in mid to High Fowler's if possible.

  Rationale: To facilitate feeding and prevent aspiration.

- Place a towel or protective cover over the client's chest.

- Check to be sure that the name on the tray corresponds with the client's name and that food in the tray is consistent with the ordered dietary and special needs.

- Position yourself at the client's eye level.

- Place the tray on the side that the patient can see and access.

- Allow the client adequate time to eat at his or her own pace.

# BASIC NURSING SKILLS

## TERMS TO REMEMBER:

- **Vital signs**: Basic measurements of body's functions.

- **Blood pressure**: The pressure exerted by the blood against the walls of the blood vessels, especially the arteries.

- **Pulse**: The rhythmic dilation of an artery that results from beating of the heart. Pulse is often measured by feeling the arteries of the wrist or neck.

- **Body temperature:** The level of heat produced and sustained by the body processes.

- **Asepsis:** Absence of the microorganisms that produce sepsis or septic disease.

- **Personal Protective Equipment (PPE):** Specialized clothing or equipment worn by an employee for protection against infectious materials.

- **Hand hygiene**: Making hands clean by washing them with running water and soap or alcohol based hand rub, before and after touching anything to avoid contamination.

## SKILLS TO MASTER:

- Measuring vital signs
- Hand washing
- Use of PPE
- Dressing a client
- Shaving a client
- Transferring a client
- Ambulating a client

- Proper client positioning

- Performing range-of-motion exercises

- Assisting client with elimination needs

- Measuring intake and output

Certified Nursing Assistants provide direct client care to patients in a multitude of health-care settings. When a patient is in a medical facility, the CNA should take care of their basic health needs as well as help them to rehabilitate. This can include skills like changing bed sheets, and bathing. Other tasks include feeding patients, ensuring safety at all times, and checking vital signs.

Taking Vital Signs

CNAs are responsible for taking patients' vital signs most hospitals and other health care facilities. Vital signs are generally taken during rounds on a regular basis and are usually required to be documented on the patient's medical records.

**Normal Vital Signs:**

| | |
|---|---|
| **Neonate** | |
| Respiration | 30 – 60 breaths/minute |
| Pulse | 120 – 160 beats/minute |
| **Child 2 to 4 years** | |
| Respiration | 24 – 32 breaths/minute |
| Pulse | 90 – 130 beats/minute |
| **Child 6 to 10 years** | |
| Respiration | 15 – 26 breaths/minute |
| Pulse | 75 – 120 beats/minute |
| Blood Pressure | 80/40 – 110/60 mm Hg |
| **Neonate/Adult** | |
| Respiration | 12 – 18 breaths/minute |
| Pulse | 60 – 100 beats/minute |
| Blood Pressure | 100/60 – 140/90 mm Hg |

## BLOOD PRESSURE

CNA training courses teach techniques for checking blood pressure with both automatic pressure-reading machines and the older-style sphygmomanometer and stethoscope.

*Selecting correct blood pressure cuff:*

- To accurately measure blood pressure, choose a cuff of appropriate size. The inflatable bladder of the cuff should have:

  - Width: 40% of the upper arm circumference (about 12-14 cm in the average adult)

  - Length: 80% of upper arm circumference (almost long enough to encircle the arm)

*Preparatory pointers:*

- Avoid smoking or drinking caffeinated beverages for 30 minutes before BP is taken and rest for at least 5 minutes.

- Palpate brachial artery.

- Position arm at the level of the heart, approximately at the level of the 4$^{th}$ intercostal space at its junction with the sternum.

- If the client is seated, rest the arm on a table a little above the waist; if standing, support the arm at the mid chest level.

*Measuring blood pressure:*

- Center the BP bladder over the brachial artery. The lower border of the cuff should be about 2.5cm above the antecubital crease.

- Take the baseline BP by palpation to determine how high to raise the cuff pressure, then add 30mmHg to it.

- Place the bell of the stethoscope lightly over the brachial artery.

  Rationale: Low pitch sounds like the Korotkoff sounds in BP taking, are best heard with the bell.

- Inflate the cuff rapidly then deflate it slowly at a rate of 2 to 3 mmHg per second. Determine the systolic and diastolic pressures.

**BP Classification (Adults older than 18 years)**

| Category | Systolic (mm Hg) | Diastolic (mm Hg) |
|---|---|---|
| Normal | <120 | <80 |
| Prehypertension | 120 – 139 | 80 – 89 |
| Hypertension<br><br>Stage I<br>Stage II | <br><br>140 – 159<br>160 and above | <br><br>90 – 99<br>100 and above |

## HEART RATE

- Radial pulse is commonly used.

- With the pads of your index and middle fingers, compress the radial artery until maximum pulsation is detected.

- Count the rhythm for one full minute. In some facilities, the rate is counted for 15 seconds and multiplied by 4 if the rhythm is regular. If the rhythm is unusually fast or slow, then count for 60 seconds.

## TEMPERATURE

Normal Body Temperature

| Method | Celsius | Fahrenheit | Time of measurement | Pointer |
|---|---|---|---|---|
| Oral | 37.0° | 98.6° | 3 to 5 minutes | Most accessible |
| Rectal | 37.6° | 99.6° | 1 to2 minutes | Most accurate |
| Axillary | 36.5° | 97.6° | 5 to 10 minutes | Safest |

- Factors that may affect reading: elderly client, faulty thermometer, environment, infection, dehydration.

- Rectal temperatures are higher than oral temperatures by about 0.4° to 0.5°C (0.7° to 0.9°F).

- Abnormalities:

  - Fever or pyrexia: elevated body temperature.

  - Hyperpyrexia: extreme elevation in temperature, above 41.1°C (106°F).

  - Hypothermia: abnormally low temperature, below 35°C (95°F) rectally.

- When using glass thermometer, shake thermometer down to 35°C (96°F).

- Tympanic membrane temperature:

  - Make sure external auditory canal is free of cerumen.

  - Position probe into the canal and wait for 2 to 3 seconds.

## RESPIRATORY RATE

- Observe the rhythm, rate, depth and effort of breathing.

- Count number of respirations in 1 minute either by visual inspection or by listening over the client's trachea with stethoscope.

- Breathing abnormalities:

  - Tachypnea: rapid breathing.

  - Bradypnea: slowed breathing.

  - Apnea: temporary cessation of breath.

  - Dyspnea: difficult, labored or painful breathing.

  - Hyperpnea: abnormally deep breathing.

  - Hyperventilation: abnormally rapid, deep and prolonged breathing.

  - Hypoventilation: abnormally slow, shallow, and short breathing.

  - Orthopnea: inability to breathe except when on upright position.

**Maintaining Cleanliness/Asepsis**

CNA's bedside care activities often include performing duties such as bed making, changing linens, and cleaning up the client and the environment. These activities necessitate proper handling and disposal of biohazardous materials such as bodily fluids and contaminated articles. The use of asepsis and observing personal hygiene are paramount in minimizing the spread of infection.

- Alert: Determine whether aseptic technique is performed correctly. Use appropriate supplies to maintain asepsis.

- Standard: Hands are washed without recontamination.

## HAND WASHING

- The most important and most basic action to prevent transmission of infection.

- Hands should be under flow of water.

- Keep hands and forearms lower than elbows.

- Use antibacterial soap. Lather and wash hands using friction for 15 seconds.

- Do not allow washed hands to touch inside of sink.

*Pointers in hand washing:*

- Stand with clothes away from the sink.

- Turn on water and adjust temperature to warm; leave water running.

- Wet wrists and hands; keep hands lower than the elbow throughout the procedure.

- Apply soap or cleansing agent and wash with friction.

- Rinse hands and wrists with fingertips pointed down.

- Dry hands with paper towel from fingertips to wrists.

- Use another dry paper towel to turnoff faucet.

- Dispose used paper towel.

## PERSONAL PROTECTIVE EQUIPMENT (PPE)

The type of PPE used can vary based on the level of precautions required. Depending on the state of the patient and their condition, you should choose a more protective PPE when necessary. The procedure for putting on and removing PPEs should be tailored to the specific type of PPE.

In many cases, you respective facility will have a set of instructions that come with it. Ensure you are familiar with them.

However, for the sake of preparation, below is the standard procedure of dawning typical PPEs.

***Sequence for putting on PPE:***

1. Gown

   - Fasten in back of neck and waist.

2. Mask or respirator

   - Secure ties or elastic bands at middle of head and neck.

   - Fit snug to face and below chin

3. Goggles or face shield

   - Place over face and eyes and adjust to fit.

4. Gloves

   - Extend to cover wrist of gown.

***Sequence for removing PPE:***

- Remove all PPE before exiting the client's room except the mask or respirator, if worn. Remove the mask or respirator after leaving the room and closing the door.

- Wash hands or use an alcohol-based hand sanitizer immediately after removing all PPE.

1. Gloves

   - Using a gloved hand, grasp the palm area of the other gloved hand and peel off the first glove.

   - Slide fingers of ungloved hand under remaining glove at wrist and peel off second glove over first glove then discard.

2. Goggles or face shield

   ▪ Remove from the back by lifting head band or ear pieces.

3. Gown

   ▪ Unfasten gown ties, taking care that sleeves don't contact your body.

   ▪ Pull gown away from neck and shoulders, touching inside of gown only.

   ▪ Turn gown inside out and discard.

4. Mask or respirator

   ▪ Grasp bottom ties or elastics of the mask, then the ones at the top, and remove without touching the front.

***What type of PPE would you wear?***

- Giving a bed bath: generally none

- Contact with oral secretions: gloves

- Transporting a client in a wheel chair: none

- Responding to an emergency where blood is spurting: gloves, fluid-resistant gown, mask, goggles/eye shield

- Spurting blood from a vein: gloves

- Cleaning incontinent client with diarrhea: gloves with or without gown

- Handling bedpan: gloves

- Exposure to wounds: gloves, gown, mask

- Taking vital signs: none

- Feeding a client: none

- Handling sharpsneedles: gloves, discard sharps, needles in the sharps/ puncture-resistant container

# BED MAKING

Hospital beds must be made up in a specific manner. Bed-making is one of the fundamental chores that every nurse aide has to perform during her career. Bed-making requirements differ based on whether the bed is occupied, if the patient is post-operative, and whether the bed is being cleaned and deodorized following a terminal client.

## Making an OCCUPIED BED

- Standard: Occupied bed must be neat and wrinkle free with client and bed placed in the appropriate positions.

- In an occupied bed, the client is on bed with the side rails up, if applicable, while the bed is being made.

- Dirty linen: A linen that contain no visible body fluids. Gloves may be worn.

- Soiled linen: A linen contaminated with body fluids. Gloves must be worn.

- At the end of the procedure, the bed must be left with side rails up if indicated.

### *Pointers in making an occupied bed:*

- Remove top linen while keeping the client covered.

- Position client on one side of the bed with side rail up.

- Tuck dirty linen under the client.

- Replace bottom linen on first side. Tuck corners and sides neatly under mattress.

- Reposition client to other side.

- Remove dirty linen by rolling together, holding away from clothing and placing dirty linen in appropriate container. Dispose gloves if used and do hand washing.

- Complete tucking linen under mattress.

- Reposition client in position of comfort.

- Place top sheet over individual. Remove dirty covering. Tuck bottom sheet corners and bottom edge under mattress.

- Spread blanket over the client then tuck under mattress. Pull top edge of sheet over top edge of blanket.

- Remove and replace pillowcase.

**Personal Care**

Assisting clients with personal care is among the primary duties of a CNA. This involves any activities of daily living the client has difficulty performing on his or her own, such as bathing, ambulating, oral care, toileting, and eating. Nurse Aides must be able to safely help the client with such tasks while allowing for optimal self-care. Refer to the previous chapter for the discussion of ADLs.

## DRESSING A CLIENT

- Standard: A client or resident is dressed in his or her own clothes, including footwear. Allow client to choose own clothing when able.

- Clothing includes undergarments, dress, or shirt or blouse and pants, socks and footwear.

## SHAVING A CLIENT

- Standard: The client should be free of facial hair without abrasions or lacerations.

*Pointers in Shaving:*

- Apply shaving cream.

- Shave while holding skin taut and using single, short strokes in the direction of hair growth and rinse razor frequently.

- Rinse face with warm cloth and apply after shave product as necessary.

- Observe precautions in using electrical equipment for electric shave.

## TRANSFERRING A CLIENT

**Transferring a Client to Wheelchair using a Transfer Belt or Gait Belt**

- Standard: Apply transfer belt, assist client to stand, pivot and sit in wheelchair with proper body alignment.

*Pointers in transferring client:*

- Lower bed to appropriate position and position wheelchair at bedside.

- Lock the brakes to prevent unnecessary movements.

- Place client in sitting position and apply transfer belt firmly around client's waist. Allow one to two fingers between belt and the waist.

- Adjust transfer belt over clothing with the buckle off the center.

- Provide client with non-skid footwear.

- Using underhand grasp, grasp transfer belt on both sides.

- Assist client to stand, pivot and sit on the wheelchair.

- Secure client's feet on the footrests.

## Transferring a Client Using Mechanical Lift

- Standard: Transfer the client safely using mechanical lift. Review facility policy for use of lift according to manufacturer's instructions.

*Pointers in transferring client:*

- Place the chair or commode at a 90-degree angle to the bed so that the nurse aide will have enough room to work.

- Place client in supine position.

- Position a sling under the client's body by rolling the client onto the sling.

- Place bed in low position and place lift over the client.

- Fasten lift's chains securely.

- Stand at the client's head and keep a hand on the part of the sling nearest the head while asking for the assistance of another aide or member of the team to operate the lift.

- Slowly move the lift to new position with the client above the next resting place and lowered slowly.

- Turn off switch and detach the chains.

**Ambulating a Client with a Transfer Belt**

- Standard: Ambulate the client safely using transfer belt.

*Pointers in ambulation:*

- Lock bed or chair wheels, if appropriate.

- Provide non-skid footwear to the client.

- Apply transfer belt firmly around the client's waist allowing one to two fingers to be slipped between belt and the client.

- Assist client to standing position while standing at the client's affected side.

- Assist the client to walk while walking to the side and slightly behind the client. Hold the transfer belt using under hand grasp.

- Encourage the client to ambulate normally with the heel striking the floor first.

## POSITIONING A CLIENT

**Placing Client in Side-Lying Position**

- Standard: Maintain proper body alignment with dependent extremities supported and bony prominences protected.

- Acceptable positions: Side-lying position or with knees flexed with padding between knees and ankles.

*Pointers in positioning the client:*

- Raise side rail on unprotected side of the bed.

- Position client on side in the center of the bed in side-lying position.

- Apply necessary padding:

  - Behind back

  - Under head

  - Between legs

- ▪ Supporting dependent arm

***Positioning a client in a chair:***

- Place feet flat against the floor.

- Position knees and hips at right angles and straighten the spine.

- Support their elbows on the arm rests.

- Place hand rolls, footrest or holsters, if needed.

## RANGE OF MOTION EXERCISES

Range of motion (ROM) exercises are used to promote flexibility and mobility.

- Standard: Perform range of motion exercises without going past the point of resistance, discomfort, or pain.

- Support body part involved and never force a joint beyond its present range of motion.

- Active ROM: These are self-ROM that a client performs on his own when he still has muscle strength to perform movements.

- Passive ROM: These are done with the assistance of the nurse aide in weaker clients.

- Ideally, exercises should be done once per day.

- Do each exercise 10 times to the point of resistance and hold for 30 seconds.

- Different range of motion movements:

  - ▪ Flexion: bending movement that decreases the angle of a joint, e.g. bending the elbow, clenching a hand into a fist.

  - ▪ Extension: straightening movement that increases the angle between two body parts, e.g. standing up.

  - ▪ Abduction: motion that pulls a body part away from the midline of the body, e.g. raising the arms up.

  - ▪ Adduction: motion that pulls a part toward the midline of the body or limb, e.g. bringing fingers together, dropping arms to the side.

- Pronation: rotational movement where the hand and the upper arm are turned inwards. Pronation of the foot refers to turning the foot outward.

- Supination: for the arms, the forearms or palms are rotated outwards. Supination of the foot refers to turning of the sole of foot inwards.

- Plantar flexion: bending foot and pointing toe downwards. Plantar means "sole of the foot."

- Dorsal flexion: bending foot upwards toward the shin. Dorsal means "top of the foot."

- Internal rotation: "medial rotation" refers to rotation towards the axis of the body.

- External rotation: "lateral rotation" refers to rotation away from the center of the body.

## ELIMINATION

### Assisting Patient who Requires Urinary Catheterization

- Drape client and expose only the perineum.

- Female client:

  - In assisting the nurse during catheterization, the client is placed on dorsal recumbent position with knees flexed or in the Sims position.

  - The catheter is secured on the client's inner thigh.

- Male client:

  - The client is placed on supine position.

  - Catheter is secured on the lower abdomen.

- Coil excess tubing flatly on bed and attach tubing to the side of the bed with a plastic catheter clamp or a rubber band and safety pin.

- Keep the drainage bag off the floor by attaching to the bed frame.

- Empty the bag at regular intervals (usually every 8 hours) so that it does not overfill and cause urine to back flow in the tubing.

### Assisting with a Bedpan

- Assist patient onto bedpan, using one of the following methods:

- Have the client lift up from a recumbent position as you push pan into position.

- Have the client assume sitting position lift up as you place pan in position.

- Roll a more immobilized client onto pan.

- Elevate head of the bed to mid or High-Fowler's position.

- Place toilet tissue and call bell within client's reach.

- Carry bedpan to the bathroom with gloves and dispose contents into the toilet.

**Measurements and Documentation**

Nursing assistants are responsible for documenting all of the care that they provide. They record any interventions, vital signs, input and output of urine or other measurements in a chart or the patient's medical record.

## CALCULATING INTAKE AND OUTPUT

Measuring fluid intake and output gives an indication of how well the kidneys are functioning. Fluid is not necessarily only what is taken by mouth but also includes intravenous fluids. Output measurement includes urine as well as captured drainage of other fluids such as blood and emesis.

- Standard: The nurse aide measures intake and output in cubic centimeters (cc) or milliliters (ml).

- Intake is any measurable fluid that goes into the patient's body.

- Output is any measurable fluid that comes from the body.

- Write down the intake and output amounts in the units of measurement.

- Convert the measured unit into the units to be recorded on the intake and output chart.

- Calculate all measured quantities listed as client intake for a time period.

- Add all the measured quantities listed as client's output for a time period.

*Conversion Table:*

| Standard unit | Equivalent to | Approximate conversion |
|---|---|---|
| 1 tablespoon | 3 teaspoons | 15 ml |
| 1 fluid ounce | 2 tablespoons | 30 ml |
| 1cup | 8 fluid ounces | 240 ml |
| 1 pint | 2cups<br><br>16 fluid ounces | 480 ml |
| 1 quart | 2 pints | 960 ml |
| 1 gallon | 4 quarts<br><br>128 fluid ounces | 3.8 l |
| 1 gallon = 4 quarts = 8 pints = 16 cups = 128 fluid ounces | | |

# RESTORATIVE SKILLS

## TERMS TO REMEMBER

- **Assistive Device:** Any device that is designed, made, or adapted to assist a person in performing a particular task. Examples of assistive devices include canes, crutches, walkers, wheelchair, and transfer belts.

- **Contracture:** An abnormal, often permanent, shortening in muscle or scar tissue, that results in distortion or deformity, especially of a joint of the body.

- **Debility:** The quality or state of being weak, feeble, or infirm; especially physical weakness.

- **Immobility:** The therapeutic or unavoidable restriction of a client's physical activity.

- **Pressure Ulcer:** *decubitus ulcer, bedsore*; A localized area of infracted tissue characterized by a reddish area that does not blanche, is warm to the touch, and leads to skin breakdown.

- **Range of Motion (ROM):** The full movement potential of a joint, usually its range of flexion and extension.

- **Rehabilitation:** Type of health care that helps a patient regain the highest possible functional state.

- **Restorative Care:** Care that focuses on helping a patient return to and maintain a level of health and well-being.

## SKILLS TO MASTER:

- Client positioning

- Performing different range of motion exercises

- Client ambulation

- Transferring a client

- Use of assistive devices

- Crutch walking gaits

- Skin care

- Assisting in personal care

Rehabilitation and restorative care cover very important aspects of health care provided to patients and residents no matter their age. Clients may get this special care in the hospital, a nursing home, an assisted living home, a rehabilitation hospital, an outpatient center, or in the client's own residence. Restorative care is a challenging area of nursing that offers so much more to the patient's quality of life. Through this health care service, the nurse aide helps a patient or resident to restore their lost abilities and to prevent further loss of ability with the end goal of promoting an optimum level of function and comfort.

Restorative skills integrate the basic principles of prevention in a holistic approach, addressing not only physiological needs but also the psychosocial concerns of a client. CNAs are trained to perform restorative activities like ambulation, client positioning, assistance in ADLs, ROM exercises, facilitating therapeutic communication, and collaborating with the client's family and other members of the health care team. The provision of such care promotes health and maintenance, prevents the occurrence or progress of diseases, and helps manage the complications of long-term debilities.

**What are the Responsibilities of the CNA?**

- Assist clients with exercises and related activities to maintain mobility and maximize independence.

- Perform routine restorative nursing care and services.

- Facilitate implementation of the client's or resident's ADL program which commonly involves personal hygiene, dressing, feeding, and elimination assistance.

- Accurately document restorative care rendered in the resident's record.

- Notify nurse-in-charge or the appropriate department of any actual or arising client's problems for the necessary interventions to be carried out.

- Monitor residents to ensure the proper use of assistive devices and provision of individualized care to address expressed needs, e.g. positioning, ambulation assistance.

- Assist in the transfer and transportation of residents as warranted.

CNAs are often confronted with concerns on immobility and its complications, including clients' compliance to therapy, comfort, and their capabilities of self-care. This section discusses selected client needs requiring rehabilitation and restorative care to help you better understand the concepts, principles, and skills involved in the abovementioned service.

## IMMOBILTY

Individuals who have inactive lifestyles or who are faced with inactivity because of illness or injury are at risk for many problems that can affect major body systems. Whether immobility causes any problems often depends on the duration of the inactivity, the client's health status, and the client's sensory awareness.

*Adverse Effects of Immobility:*

| SYSTEM | COMPLICATION |
| --- | --- |
| Integumentary | Decubitus ulcer |
| | Infection |
| Musculoskeletal | Muscle atrophy |
| | Contractures |
| | Decreased muscle mass |
| | Osteoporosis |
| | Pathologic fracture |
| | Deformities |
| | Decreased stability |
| Respiratory | Respiratory infections |
| | Pneumonia |
| | Atelectasis |
| Cardiovascular | Thrombus formation |
| | Embolism |
| | Orthostatic hypotension |

| Metabolic | Decreased metabolic rate |
| | Anorexia |
| | Weight loss |
| | Slow wound healing and tissue growth |
| | Fluid and electrolyte imbalances |
| Elimination | Constipation |
| | Urinary stasis |
| | Urinary tract infection |
| | Renal calculi/stones |
| Psychosocial | Depression |
| | Sensory deprivation |
| | Confusion |
| | Dependence |
| | Insomnia |
| | Restlessness |

## Rehabilitation Principles of Mobility

**1. Positioning**: A client or resident on bed should be repositioned every two hours unless contraindicated. Different positions also correspond to specific physiologic purposes.

| POSITION | FUNCTION |
| --- | --- |
| Flat/supine | Minimizes hip flexion |
| Side-lying, side with leg bent | Promote drainage of secretions and prevent aspiration |
| Fowler's/head elevated | Maximal lung expansion |
| Head and knees slightly elevated | Increases venous return |
| | Alleviates pressure on lumbosacral area |

| Modified Trendelenburg (Feet elevated 20° and head slightly elevated/shock position) | Increases venous return<br><br>Increases blood flow to the brain |
|---|---|
| Elevation of extremity | Promotes venous return |
| Lithotomy (flat on back, thighs flexed, legs abducted) | Exposes perineum |
| Prone | Promotes extension of hip joints |

**2. Exercises**: When people are ill, they may need to perform ROM exercise until they can regain their normal activity levels.

- Performing ROM improves circulation, muscle tone and strength, joint mobility and prevents contractures, disuse syndrome, atrophy, and bone loss.

*Types of Exercises:*

| EXERCISE | DESCRIPTION | PURPOSE |
|---|---|---|
| Passive Range of Motion (PROM) | Performed by the CNA without assistance from client | Promote circulation;<br><br>Improve joint range of motion |
| Active Assistive Range of Motion | Performed by the client with assistance from the CNA | Measures and promotes motion in the joint and limbs |
| Active Range of Motion | Performed by the client without assistance | Maintains joint mobility |
| Active Resistive Range of Motion | Performed by the client against resistance | Use of resistance increases muscle strength, power and tone;<br><br>Use 5-lb sand bags/weights |
| Isometric Exercises | Performed by client;<br><br>Instruct client to alternate contraction and relaxation of muscle without moving joint | Maintains muscle strength |
| Isotonic Exercises | Performed actively by the client;<br><br>Contraction, tension remains unchanged and the muscle's length changes | Increases muscle strength and tone |

*Procedural Guidelines:*

- Lock wheels of bed, lower head of bed and assist resident to lie on back, without pillow and in good alignment as able.

- Cover resident with bath blanket or top sheet and uncover only the part being exercised.

- ROM exercise for shoulders:

  - Begin with arm straight at side while supporting the elbow and wrist.

  - Move straight arm out at a right angle to body then return to side.

- ROM exercise for elbows:

  - Bend elbow moving hand toward shoulder, then straighten the arm.

- ROM exercise for forearms:

  - Begin with arm flat on bed. Turn hand with palm up, then turn palm downward.

- ROM exercise for wrists:

  - Begin with palm up. Bend hand down, then straighten hand.

  - Bend hand up, then straighten hand.

  - Turn hand toward thumb, then turn hand toward little finger.

- ROM exercise for hands:

  - Put your fingers over resident's finger. Curl fingers to form a fist, then straighten fingers.

  - Touch resident's thumb to each finger.

- ROM exercise for hips and knees:

  - Begin with leg straight, supporting leg with one hand under knee and one hand under ankle.

  - Bend knee and slowly raise the leg, then straighten the knee and lower the leg.

  - Move straight leg away from the center of the body, then back to center.

  - Turn leg inward then outward.

- ROM exercise for ankle and feet:

  - Move forefoot in a circle clockwise the counter-clockwise.

- ROM exercise for toes and feet:

  - Curl toes downward then straightened.

  - Move each toe away from the middle toe, then vice versa.

**3. Ambulation:**

- *Use of Tilt Table:*

  - Weight bearing on long bones to prevent decalcification.

  - Use elastic stockings to prevent postural hypotension.

  - Check blood pressure.

  - Stop procedure when client experiences decrease in BP, dizziness, pallor, diaphoresis, tachycardia and nausea.

- *Transferring Client*: Many clients require some assistance in transferring between bed and chair or wheelchair, between wheelchair and toilet, and between bed and stretcher.

  - For a client with a stronger and a weaker side, move him or her toward the stronger side.

    Rationale: This will make it easier for the client to pull the weak side.

  - Move the client with the drawsheet. Sliding the patient across a surface predisposes skin breakdown or irritation.

  - During the transfer, explain step by step what the client should do, for example, "Move your right foot forward."

  - Transfer (walking) belts provide the greatest safety.

  - Because wheelchairs and stretchers are unstable, they can predispose the client to falls and injury.

  - Note: *Practice Guidelines for Wheelchair Safety:*

    o Always lock the brakes on both wheels when the client transfers in and out of it.

- o Lower footplates after transfer, and place client's feet on them

    - o Use seat belts that fasten behind the wheelchair to protect confused clients from falls.

    - o Back the wheelchair into or out of an elevator, rear wheels first.

- Sitting Client at the Edge of Bed:

    - Place hand under knees and shoulders of the client.

    - Instruct client to push elbow into bed while lifting shoulders and bringing legs over edge of the bed.

- Assisting Client to Stand:

    - Face client and grasp each side of rib cage.

    - Push your knee against one knee of the client.

    - Rock client forward as he or she stands ensuring that the knees are locked while standing.

    - Pivot with client to position and transfer client's weight quickly to chair on his or her stronger side.

- Crutch Walking:

    - Weight should be supported on the handpiece, not in the axilla.

    - Rationale: Weight bearing on the axilla leads to damage of the brachial plexus nerve.

    - Position crutches 6 to 8 inches to side of the leg.

    - Reinforce teachings on how to perform the needed crutch walking gaits:

*Crutch Walking Gaits:*

| Gait | Indication | Steps |
|------|-----------|-------|
| Four-point Gait | Minimal weight bearing allowed on both feet | Right crutch, left foot, left crutch, right foot |
| Two-point Gait | More stable than four-point gait; weight-bearing allowed on both feet | Advance right crutch and left foot together; then left crutch and right foot together |

| Three-point Gait | Weight-bearing is allowed only on one leg | Advance weak leg and both crutches simultaneously; advance good leg |
|---|---|---|
| Swing-to Gait | Partial weight-bearing allowed on both legs; | Advance both crutches, then leg or both feet at the level of the crutches |
| Swing-through Gait | post amputation | Advance both crutches, then leg or both feet beyond the level of the crutches |

- **Alert**: For going up and down stairs, remember, "Up with the good, down with the bad," or "The good goes to heaven, the bad goes to hell."

  **Going upstairs:** Good leg, crutches, affected leg.

  **Going downstairs:** Crutches with affected leg, followed by the good leg.

*General Guidelines for Immobility:*

- Provide psychosocial support
  - Allow use of communication channels, e.g. social media, telephone.
  - Arrange schedules to accommodate visitors.
  - Provide diversional activities.
  - Encourage expression of feelings and concerns.
- Assist client with self-care
  - Start with simple, gross activity before performing more complex motions.
  - Provide feedback and acknowledge client's progress.
- Prevention of muscle contractures
  - Periodic repositioning of client.
  - Use proper body alignment and provide supportive pillows and rolls.
  - Maintain balanced diet.
- Prevention of constipation

- Ambulate client as tolerated.

- Increase fluid intake and fiber in the diet.

- Prevention of urinary stasis, UTI, and renal stones

  - Encourage regular voiding.

  - Increase fluid intake.

  - Provide indicated diet of low calcium and acid ash to acidify urine and prevent infection or calcium stone formation.

- Prevention of thrombus formation

  - Leg exercises unless contraindicated.

  - Avoid gatching bed or knee flexed position for prolonged period.

- Prevention of respiratory complications

  - Reinforce teachings on importance of positioning, coughing, and deep breathing.

- Prevention of pressure ulcers

  - Reposition client frequently, every two hours.

  - Use drawsheet when moving client on bed to avoid shearing force against the skin.

  - Assist with indicated nutrition: adequate protein, vitamins (Vitamin C), and minerals.

  - Use air mattress, flotation pads, elbow and heel pads, sheepskin.

*Stages of Pressure Ulcer:*

| Stage | Description |
| --- | --- |
| Stage I | • Intact skin<br>• Reddish area that does not blanche with pressure |
| Stage II | • Non-intact skin<br>• Partial-thickness skin loss of the epidermis and dermis<br>• Superficial ulcer resembling abrasion, blister or shallow crater |
| Stage III | • Full-thickness skin loss<br>• Damage up to subcutaneous tissues<br>• Ulcer appears as deep crater |
| Stage IV | • Full-thickness skin loss with extensive tissue destruction of muscles, bone and supporting structures<br>• Undermining and sinus tracts or tunnels may develop |

# EMOTIONAL AND MENTAL HEALTH NEEDS

## TERMS TO REMEMBER:

- **Empathy:** The ability to experience the feelings of another person. It goes beyond sympathy, which is caring and understanding for the suffering of others.

- **Mental Health**: A state of well-being in which a person is able to cope with the normal stresses of daily life and realize his or her potential (WHO, 2005).

- **Mental Hygiene**: The science that deals with measures to promote mental health, prevent mental illness and suffering, and facilitate rehabilitation of the client.

- **Mental Ill Health**: State of imbalance characterized by a disturbance in a person's thoughts, feelings, and behavior.

- **Self-concept**: Encompasses all beliefs, convictions, and ideas that constitute an individual's knowledge of himself or herself and influence his or her relationship with others.

- **Self-esteem:** An individual's personal judgment of his or her own worth obtained by analyzing how well his or her behavior conforms to his or her self-ideal.

- **Self-ideal**: An individual's perception of how he or she should behave based on certain personal standards.

- **Therapeutic Relationship**: *therapeutic alliance*. The relationship between a health care professional and a client (or patient). It is the means by which a therapist and a client hope to engage with each other, and effect beneficial change in the client.

## SKILLS TO MASTER:

- Performing mental status observation

- Maintaining a therapeutic environment

- Empathic active listening

- Assisting with personal care

- Promoting environmental safety

- Use of therapeutic communication

- Facilitating grieving process

- Encouraging verbalization or expression of needs

- Coordinating with the health care team for referral and safety measures

- Organizing occupational therapy activities

It is difficult to define the mental health of a client without considering the aspects of society or his or her environment. An individual is considered mentally fit when he or she is able to deal with societal aspects, cope with demands, and follow the expected norms of a society. Hence, psychosocial is one's psychological development in, and interaction with, a social environment.

Problems that arise with a person's psychosocial functioning can be referred to as "psychosocial dysfunction," the lack of development of the psychosocial self, often occurring alongside other dysfunctions that may be physical, emotional, or cognitive in nature. In providing comprehensive individualized quality care, CNAs not only address the physiological needs of the clients or residents, but also integrate psychosocial skills to contribute to their clients' well-being.

Alert: A healthy self-concept (e.g. positive self-esteem) is essential to psychological well-being. It is universal.

Factors affecting a person's psychosocial integrity related to ineffective coping and maladaptation include the aging process, illnesses, injuries, developmental and situational crises, losses, and the concept of death and dying. As therapeutic members of the health care team, CNAs need to have an in-depth understanding of themselves, with the self as the tool in a therapeutic relationship, and a clear grasp of the principles and skills in promoting the emotional and mental health of their clients.

## HUMAN BEHAVIOR:

What motivates human behavior? According to humanist psychologist Abraham Maslow, a person's actions are motivated in order to achieve certain needs. In their hierarchy of needs, people are motivated to fulfill basic needs before moving on to more advanced needs. People have an inborn desire to be self-actualized, to be all they can be. In order to achieve this however, a number of more basic needs must be met first, such as food, safety, love, and self-esteem.

As a client progresses up the pyramid of needs, succeeding needs become increasingly psychological and social in nature. Soon, the need for love, friendship, and intimacy become significant – followed by personal esteem and feelings of accomplishment.

*Maslow's Hierarchy of Human Needs*

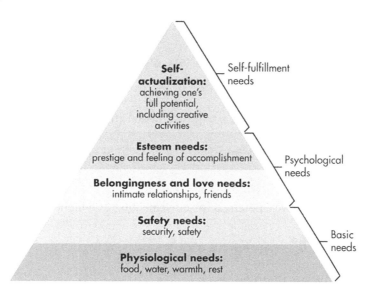

Note: CNAs facilitate the fulfillment of their clients' or residents' psychosocial needs by helping them meet the basic or lower needs first, and then progressing to the higher classifications of human needs. It is implied that clients cannot achieve emotional and mental stability without first addressing the basic physiological survival requirements. Hence, the functions of CNAs are interrelated with the physical personal care of the client with the social interactions, adaptation to stress, support system, and the therapeutic interventions of the entire team in promoting his well-being.

### Principles of Care in Mental Health:

- The client is a unique human being who needs to be accepted as a person with worth and dignity.

- The client is viewed as a holistic being with interrelated and interdependent needs. Any imbalance in one aspect of the client's personality affects the overall functioning.

- Focus on the client's strengths and potentials in planning and rendering care.

- Therapeutic relationships are the core intervention.

- Accept and respect people as individuals and strive to separate the person from any abhorrent behavior.

- Limit or reject inappropriate behavior without rejecting the individual.

- All behaviors have meaning and are meeting the needs of the person regardless of how distorted or meaningless they appear to others.

- Accept the dependency needs of the client while supporting and encouraging moves toward independence; build on the ego strengths.

- Help clients set appropriate limits for themselves or set limits for them when they are unable to do so.

- Encourage client to express feelings in a non-judgmental atmosphere.

- Recognize that client frequently responds to the behavioral expectations of others: family, peers, and the staff.

- Recognize that all clients have a potential for movement toward higher levels of emotional health.

## THERAPEUTIC RELATIONSHIP

*Roles of the CNA in a Therapeutic Relationship:*

| Role | Description |
|------|-------------|
| Facilitator of a therapeutic environment | Providing a warm, home-like, accepting atmosphere |
| Socializing agent | Improving social relationships of clients with other people by helping them develop feelings of security with others as they participate in activities |
| Counselor | Help the client understand what is happening to him/her through:<br>• Empathic listening<br>• Providing assurance as appropriate<br>• Finding acceptable outlets of anxiety |
| Teacher | Enabling client to learn more adaptive ways of coping with problems |
| Parent surrogate | Acting as a substitute parental figure |

| Care-giver | Providing personal care |
| Role model | Serving as a mature model of good mental health |

Alert: The most important skill in a therapeutic relationship is LISTENING.

### Phases of Therapeutic Relationship with the Client

| Phase | Description | Characteristics and tasks |
|---|---|---|
| Preinteraction | Begins before the initial contact with the client | • Self-exploration regarding misconceptions and prejudices of others and acknowledging one's own feelings, fears, personal values and attitudes<br><br>• SELF-AWARENESS is the main task before one can establish mutuality |
| Orientation or introductory | Initial interaction with the client | • Task: establish trust<br><br>• Assumption of the role of a stranger<br><br>• Setting expectations<br><br>• The client is never pushed to discuss areas of concern that are upsetting to him or her. |
| Working | The CNA and the client discuss and address areas of concern | • Identified needs are addressed or resolved<br><br>• Most therapeutic phase<br><br>• New adaptive behaviors are learned |
| Termination | End of the relationship | • Expression of feelings<br><br>• Learned adaptive behaviors are reinforced<br><br>• Goals and objectives are reviewed and summarized<br><br>• Referral as needed |

### Dealing with Client's Behavior During Interaction

| If the client is: | The focus of interaction should be: |
|---|---|
| Withdrawn | Non-verbal behavior |
| Depressed | Eliciting possible client's suicidal plans |

| Aggressive | Setting limits |
|---|---|
| Delusional | Not challenging the delusion directly |
| Confused | Reorient to reality or to the three spheres: time, person, place |
| Manipulative | Setting limits |
| Hyperactive | Setting limits |
| Combative | Setting limits and employing necessary security assistance |

## SECURITY NEEDS

These include needs for safety and security. Security needs are important for survival, but they are not as demanding as the physiological needs. Examples of security needs include a desire for steady employment, health care, safe neighborhoods, and shelter from the environment.

- Develop trusting relationships with the client or resident.

- Provide safe care in performing necessary procedures.

- Perform care in an organized, consistent, and confident manner.

- Answer call signals promptly and be available to help client or resident in need.

- Check in on client or resident and offer assistance even before he or she asks for help.

- Follow through on any promises you make.

- Alert: Maintaining consistency fosters trust and sense of security.

## LOVE AND SOCIAL NEEDS

These include needs for belonging, love, and affection. Maslow described these needs as less basic than physiological and security needs. Relationships such as friendships, romantic attachments, and families help fulfill this need for companionship and acceptance, as does involvement in social, community, or religious groups.

*Pointers in Assisting Client or Resident with Love and Social Needs*

For some clients or residents, you may be considered a major social contact and source of assistance in accessing contact with others.

- Listen carefully and express genuine interest in the client's or resident's concerns and activities.

- Encourage and assist client to maintain open communication and relationship with significant others.

- Determine the client's or resident's interest and find related social activities to advance this.

- Collaborate with the charge nurse, social worker, activity director, restorative team to meet social needs as appropriate.

- Arrange activities and environment to promote socialization and avoid conflicts between clients or residents.

- Never coerce a client or resident to participate in activities against his or her wishes.

- Arrange client's or resident's schedule and prepare them to be on time for social activities.

## CLIENT'S SELF CONCEPT

Alert: Promoting a positive self-concept is basic to all emotional and mental health interventions. In answering questions, look for options that focus on this concept; acknowledging the client as a person is an example.

### Client's behaviors with Low Self-Esteem:

- Self-derision and self-criticism: The client or resident may describe himself or herself as stupid, worthless, a burden, or a loser.

- Self-diminution: With feelings of powerlessness, the client minimizes his or her own abilities.

- Guilt and incessant worrying.

- Procrastination and denying pleasure.

- Altered interpersonal relationships with the health care team and significant others.

- Self-destructiveness.

- Boredom.

- Pessimism.

*Therapeutic approaches:*

- Expand the client's self-awareness

  - Use an open, trusting relationship

  - Work on the current strengths of the client

  - Maximize client's participation

- Promote client's self-exploration

  - Encourage client to accept his or her own feelings and thoughts

  - Use self-disclosure as appropriate

  - Communicate empathically, not sympathetically

  - Explore with client maladaptive thinking like:

    o Catastrophizing: thinking and expecting worst things will happen.

    o Minimizing and maximizing: minimizing positive thoughts and maximizing negative responses.

    o Black- and white- thinking: looking at situations in extremes, with no middle ground.

    o Overgeneralization: what happened once will happen again. The behavior of one is the behavior of all.

- Facilitate client's self-evaluation

  - Encourage client or resident to define and identify the problem

  - Help client identify irrational beliefs like:

    o "I must do good to be loved by everybody."

    o "I should not make any mistakes."

    o "I should agree all the time for nurses and doctors to take care of me."

    o "My whole life is a mess. There's no way out. There's no use for this therapy."

## ALTERATION IN BODY IMAGE

*Kinds of body image disturbances:*

- Changes in body size, shape, and appearance, e.g. pregnancy, weight gain or weight loss.

- Illness causing changes in structure or function of one's body, e.g. cancer, Parkinson's, leprosy.

- Failure of the body part to function properly, e.g. stroke, paralysis.

- Developmental related physical changes, e.g. adolescence, aging.

- Threatening therapeutic or medical procedures, e.g. chemotherapy, surgery, amputation.

*Principles of Body Image Disturbance*

- Abrupt significant body image changes, handicaps, are far more traumatic than those that develop gradually.

- The location of the disease or injury greatly affects the emotional response of the client: internal diseases are generally less threatening than external diseases, e.g. trauma, disfigurement.

- Changes in the genitals or breasts are perceived as a great threat and reawaken fears about sexuality and virility.

*Four Phases of Alterations of Body Image*

1. Impact phase:

   - Despair, discouragement, passive acceptance

   - Often projects guilt and anger to others

   - Sense of failure

2. Retreat phase:

   - Client becomes aware of the injury, disease, loss, or disfigurement

   - Regression behaviors

3. Acknowledgment phase:

   - Mourning or grieving for the loss

4. Reconstruction phase:

- Adapts to changes in body image

- Encouraged to try new approaches in life

### *Pointers in Specific Situations of Altered Body Image*

- **Obesity:** Weight exceeds 20% above the normal range for age, sex, and height

  - Reinforce indicated behavior modification programs, e.g. weight loss program

  - Unconditional acceptance of the client

  - Encourage realistic exercise program and coordinate long-range nutritional counseling

- **Stroke:** Problems with paralysis, loss of bowel and bladder control, speech and cognitive skills

  - Encourage speech efforts, e.g. speaking slowly, clarifying statements, providing other communication tools

  - Assist in self-care

  - Provide tactile stimulation to affected paralyzed body part

- **Amputation:** Phantom limb pain, feelings of loss, impaired role performance

  - Check client's complaint of pain, provide diversional activities and refer as necessary for pain management

  - Assist family members to work through their feelings and to accept the client as a whole person

  - Assist the client with ambulation with the use of appropriate assistive devices

- **Pregnancy:** Marked changes in a woman's body

  - Explanation and reassurance of the normal physiological changes in pregnancy

  - Encourage verbalization of feelings

  - Involve husband or significant others in the care

- **Cancer:** Emaciation, alopecia due to chemotherapy, loss of body part from surgery

- Provide skin care, wigs, and turban

- Provide conducive environment for rest and to improve the client's appetite during meals

- Involve family members in the client's personal care

- Allow the client to verbalize concerns and fears

- **Enterostomal Surgery:** Shock at initial sight, fear of fecal diversion, rejection

    - Reinforce doctor's and nurse's preoperative explanation by use of drawings, models or pictures of how stoma will appear

    - Encourage discussion and recognition of the importance of involving a "successful ostomate" in talking with the client to share experiences

- **Aging:** Aging not only causes changes in appearance but also in the resident's self-concept, abilities to perform self-care and independence

    - Note: The use of wheelchairs, canes, walkers, hearing aids, or any combination of these will have an impact on the self-esteem of the older client.

    - Allow ample time to gather information and communicate with older clients because they are often starved for someone to listen to them.

## HUMAN SEXUALITY

Human sexuality refers to the expression of sexual sensation and related intimacy between human beings, as well as the expression of identity through sex and as influenced by or based on sex. It comprises a broad range of behaviors and processes, including physiological, psychological, social, cultural, political, and spiritual or religious aspects. Sexuality needs are deeply personal, and clients may find difficulty in expressing related concerns. Personal values and barriers on the part of the CNA can also impact effective approaches in addressing these needs.

*Principles of Sexuality:*

- Human sexuality is best understood when approached holistically.

- Hospitalization alters a client's concept of self as a sexual being.

- Sexual role identity may be altered during illness.

- Cultural factors influence the client's expression of sexuality. Hospitalized clients may act out sexually to test the response of others to their sexuality, to gain control of a situation, or to gain attention.

- Sexual desire does not necessarily decrease with aging, but may be affected by age-related diseases.

- Sexual needs must be dealt with according to the developmental stage of a client.

- CNAs play a key role in sex-health education. You have to be aware of your own attitudes toward sex to respond helpfully to clients.

- Clients or residents have the right to express their sexual feelings. They should be given opportunities for this in a socially acceptable manner.

*Effects of Illness on Sexuality:*

- Depression decreases libido.

- Sexual preoccupation and abnormal expressions may be experienced by patients with psychosis.

- Some medications may cause sexual dysfunction, failure of orgasm in women and erectile or ejaculation problems in men.

- Clients with spinal cord injuries and neurological problems may lose sexual functioning.

*Aging Process and Sexuality:*

- Menopause in women: decreased estrogen supply results in decreased vaginal lubrication, shrinkage and loss of vaginal elasticity, and decreased breast size.

- Andropause in men: decreased testosterone, decreased spermatogenesis, and a longer time to achieve erection along with decreased firmness of erection.

- Prolonged abstinence from sexual activity may lead to sexual disuse syndrome.

*Guidelines in Assisting Clients with Sexual Needs:*

- Use praise and touch as appropriate to help meet needs for love and caring.

- Assist client or resident to feel good about his or her physical appearance by:

  - Providing care with occasional grooming such as new hairstyle.

- Being generous with compliments, e.g. "You look good today," or "You have beautiful blue eyes."

- Provide privacy for appropriate sexual behavior of client, e.g. knocking before entering, closing the door.

- Manage inappropriate sexual behaviors or advances:

  o Calmly direct resident to a private place following instructions of the nurse-in-charge and as indicated in the care plan.

  o Frankly and clearly confront unacceptable sexual behaviors.

  o Firmly state objection to unwanted sexual advances of a client or resident toward you or another resident.

  o Be direct and specific in informing a client or resident to stop an unwanted behavior, like "I need you to remove your hand from my breast immediately. Your behavior is unacceptable."

  o Clarify and reiterate professional roles with the client.

  o Violations of etiquette related to sexuality need to be reported immediately for your safety and the safety of other clients or residents in the area.

# CONCEPT OF LOSS AND END-OF-LIFE CARE

Death remains a great mystery. Even though dying is a natural part of existence, we tend to view death as a feared enemy. It is human nature to try to avoid things we fear. Our own fears and personal concept of death may serve as a barrier in providing care to our clients confronted with loss, death, dying and grieving process. To be therapeutic in the end-of-life care, we must have deeper awareness and acceptance of our own concept of death.

When dealing with clients and their families in situations related to loss, death, and dying, there are no exact words that can be used to alleviate their suffering. To facilitate grieving, we bring in our self as a tool in the process with the use of principles in establishing therapeutic relationships.

Alert: Check on the coping mechanisms of client and family, assist client to adjust to role changes, provide emotional support, and continuously monitor the client's response to the situation.

- The concept of loss includes both biological and physiological aspects. Components cover death, dying, grief and mourning.

  - Death: represents finality, the end of one's biological being

  - Dying: the social process of organizing activities in preparation for death

  - Grief: the sequence of subjective states following loss and accompanying mourning

  - Mourning: psychological processes that are aroused by the loss of a loved object or person

  - Disenfranchised grief: loss that is not and cannot be openly expressed and acknowledged by others. E.g. miscarriage, birth of a disabled child, death of an ex-spouse, death of a pet.

- Note: The main focus of care in a terminally ill or dying client is protection of his or her rights and meeting the needs of the client and significant others.

*Characteristic Stages (Kubler-Ross' Stages of Dying)*

| Death and dying | Grief | Description | Statement |
|---|---|---|---|
| D – Denial | Shock and disbelief | Refusal to believe the occurrence of a loss | "No, it's not me!" |
| A – Anger | Developing awareness | Emotional outburst that serves to resist the loss | "Why me?" |
| B – Bargaining | | Attempt to postpone the reality of the loss | "It's me but…if only…" |
| D – Depression | | Loneliness and interpersonal withdrawal | silence |
| A – Acceptance | Restitution or resolution of loss | Acceptance of the reality of the loss | "Yes, it's me." "I'm devoid of feelings." |

- A feeling of numbness is typical of the depression stage when the client feels a great sense of loss. It is also characterized by stoicism and grief.

- Encourage expression of loss and pain.

- The anger stage includes feelings of rage, envy, and resentment, and may be directed to the CNA other members of the team. Don't take the behavior personally.

- Statements made by the client and significant others related to grief must be acknowledged, accepted, and dealt with with compassion.

- A terminally ill or dying client responds to those around him or her with feelings of isolation.

- One of the major responsibilities in assisting a client to a peaceful death is helping meet needs for dignity, security, and self-worth.

## ASSISTING CLIENT'S WITH SPECIFIC BEHAVIORAL PROBLEMS

*Clients with Sleep Problems*

- Determine cause of sleep disturbances, which may include environmental disruptions, anxiety, pain, disruption in routines, intake of substances and elimination problems.

- Promote sleep by providing backrub, minimizing noise, and dimming lights.

- Provide reassurance and comfort measures for anxious clients.

- Orient client to environment.

- Avoid naps in the afternoon of client has difficulty sleeping at night.

- Reduce fluid intake at bed time.

## *Assisting Demanding Clients*

- Talk to the client or resident to determine the nature of the complaint or demand and report objective observations to the nurse-in-charge.

- If complaint or demand is justified, facilitate activities to correct or address the demand according to your practice or as instructed by the charge nurse.

- For unjustified complaints or demands:

  - Assure the client or resident that the complaint was heard and reported to the nurse

  - Be a good listener

  - If complaints are related to care, remain neutral, avoid being defensive or taking sides

  - Allow client or resident as much control over ADLs as allowed

  - Engage client with acceptable activities of his or her interest

  - Check for possible causes of unjustified complaints such as boredom, pain, anger, need for attention, and other unmet needs.

## *Assisting Verbally or Physically Aggressive Clients*

- Look for underlying causes of the behavior.

- Follow instructions of the charge nurse and behavior management plan as appropriate.

- Yelling or Screaming Client:

  - Distract client with a snack, an object of interest, or with a discussion of a topic he or she wants.

- Verbal Aggression: This includes arguing, threatening, or accusing, usually in a loud and angry voice.

- Physical Aggression: Combative behavior that may include fighting.

- Remain calm, reassuring and use non-threatening body language.

- Do not be defensive. Do not argue or try to reason with the client.

- Move the resident or client into a private space.

  - For an attack directed at you, leave safely or request assistance of a caregiver to calm the resident.

  - For an attack directed at another resident, request assistance and remove both the residents to separate quiet areas.

- Safety precautions for physical aggression:

  - Notify charge nurse quietly but promptly, and obtain needed assistance

  - Protect yourself with padding, as needed as per facility policy

  - Take threats seriously and maintain distance

  - Do not try to touch or turn your back on the combative client or resident.

  - Don't back a client or resident into a corner, especially if the fight is related to space.

- Follow guidelines in the application of restraints if ordered.

### Assisting Clients with Cognitive Impairment

Neurological disorders like CVA and traumatic brain injuries, or age-related cognitive disorders such as Alzheimer's or Parkinson's diseases, significantly impair the cognitive abilities of a client. Impaired cognitive abilities directly result in altered decision making, slowed mental capacity, alterations on perceptions, memories, behavioral responses, self-determination, and capacity to self-care.

### Pointers in Cognitive Impairment:

- Organic mental disorders: main characteristic is a psychological or behavioral abnormality associated with transient or permanent dysfunction of the brain.

- Delirium: a syndrome that usually develops over a short period of time. Manifestations affecting sensorium fluctuate and are often reversible and temporary.

- Dementia: A syndrome characterized by loss of intellectual abilities to such extent that social and occupational functions are negatively affected. Often, the disorders are progressive and follow an irreversible course in which the damage remains permanent.

  - **3 Ps for dementia care**:

    o **P**rotecting dignity

    o **P**reserving function

    o **P**romoting quality of life

  - Memory impairment of dementia, e.g. Alzheimer's, include:

    o **J** – judgment

    o **A** – affect

    o **M** – memory

    o **C** – confusion

    o **O**– orientation

- Geriatric Alerts:

  - The cardinal rule is not to push too fast in getting information, assisting with ADLs, or insisting that the person socialize. Continued pressure and insistence on a task may result in combative behavior.

  - Orient client to reality and monitor activities of confused client.

- Geriatric priority:

  - Situations that can lead to combative behavior are threats to self-image, e.g. new things or people in the environment, illusions, pressure to remember and direct confrontation.

  - **3 Rs: Routine, Reinforcement, Repetition** – key aspects of care.

  - **Reminiscence and life review** help the client resume progression through the grief process associated with disappointing life events and increase self-esteem as successes are reviewed.

- Provide a quiet, structured environment to increase consistency and promote feelings of security

  - Avoid dependency.

  - Establish routine for ADLs.

  - Do not isolate client from other residents in the unit.

  - Provide assistive devices and handrails.

  - Do not change schedules suddenly.

- Promote contact with reality

  - Make brief and frequent contact.

  - Give feedback.

  - Use concrete ideas in communication.

  - Orient client frequently to reality and environment. Allow him or her to have familiar personal items with him or her. Use clocks, calendars, and daily schedules.

  - Use simple explanations and face-to-face interaction. Do not shout.

  - Allow client sufficient time to complete tasks.

- Provide diversion activities that enhance self-esteem

  - Recognize specific accomplishments.

  - Maintain a structured yet flexible schedule to prevent boredom.

  - Devise methods for memory deficits:

    - Name sign and picture of the client on the door

    - Identifying sign on the outside of the door for specific areas, like dining room

    - Large clock, with oversize numbers and hands

    - Large calendar, indicating one day at a time, with month, day and year in bold print

# SPIRITUAL AND CULTURAL NEEDS

## TERMS TO REMEMBER:

- **Culture:** The sum of attitudes, customs, and beliefs that distinguishes one group of people from another.

- **Cultural Diversity:** The variety of human societies or cultures in a specific region, or in the world as a whole.

- **Customs:** Traditional practices or usual ways of doing something followed by a social group or people.

- **Faith:** The confidence or trust in a being, object, living organism, deity, view, or in the doctrines or teachings of a religion.

- **Ethnicity:** A socially-defined category of people who identify with each other based on common ancestral, social, cultural, or national experience.

- **Ethnocentrism:** Judging another culture solely by the values and standards of one's own culture.

- **Religion:** An organized collection of beliefs, cultural systems, and world views that relate humanity to an order of existence.

- **Spirituality:** The essence of the human being that transcends and connects him to God or the Divine power.

- **Spiritual Distress:** A state in which an individual's relationship to God or other higher force is impaired and/or spiritual needs cannot be fulfilled.

- **Transcultural Care:** A humanistic and scientific approach and practice that focuses on how patterns of behavior in illness, health, and caring are influenced by the values and beliefs of specific cultural groups.

## SKILLS TO MASTER:

- Assessing different spiritual needs

- Assisting client in spiritual distress

- Using therapeutic communication

- Understanding one's and client's faith

- Differentiating the diversities in beliefs and practices

- Collaborating with client's support group or support system

- Providing culture specific care

- Providing spiritual milieu

## SPIRITUALITY

Most people are confronted with the belief that they have a connection with a power greater than themselves. A positive, harmonious relationship with God or a higher power or being helps clients feel unified with other people and with nature. It fosters love and worth despite their imperfections, errors, and suffering. People are filled with joy, hope, peace, and purpose when they transcend beyond themselves. Spirituality can help clients who are experiencing pain, loss, suffering, or who are having difficulties finding meaning in these experiences develop more strength to face life's challenges.

Spirituality is the essence of our being that transcends and connects us to God or to that Divine power and other beings. It is not synonymous with religion. Spirituality is a more general term that includes religion but also encompasses the general human impulse to reach out toward the greater whole of which we all are a part. The difference between religion and spirituality is simply that most religions offer a specific set of beliefs and structures to help people realize their innate spirituality. Religion could be viewed as a significant expression of spirituality, but highly spiritual individuals may not necessarily identify with a specific religion.

The sense of fulfillment or completeness meets the highest level of human needs; self-actualization. Failure to meet this need leads to hopelessness or spiritual distress. CNAs can help clients or residents bridge the gap in their spirituality by employing principles that support their clients' spiritual interests.

## SPIRITUAL NEEDS

All individuals have recognized, expressed, or even unacknowledged spiritual needs. Some of these needs become more pronounced later in life or during periods of illness and when facing difficult realities in life, like crises or death.

- **Love**: The most important spiritual need.

  - People need to feel that they are cared about and can offer caring feelings.

  - Spiritual love is "unconditional" – it is given unselfishly regardless of one's background, personality, and condition.

- **Meaning and Purpose**

  - The final developmental task of aging and in self-actualization is having a sense of integrity.

  - Integrity also holds on to the belief that all life experiences, whether bad or good, have meaning and purpose. Some clients may believe that their suffering and sorrow have eternal purpose or allow God to be glorified.

- **Hope**: Hope is an optimistic attitude of mind based on an expectation of positive outcomes related to events and circumstances in one's life.

  - For clients or residents, hope propels them to face the future in the presence of pain and suffering, because they believe relief and eternal reward are possible.

- **Dignity**: Every individual has an innate worth regardless of their appearance, function, and productivity.

  - When clients lack the attributes that command dignity in their community or according to the norms of a society, value and worth can be derived through their connection to God.

- **Forgiveness**: The process of ceasing to feel resentment, indignation, or anger for a perceived offense, and ceasing to demand punishment or restitution.

  - Carrying the burden of the mistakes committed by or to the clients is significantly stressful and may pose detrimental effects on their health.

  - Lack of forgiveness robs a person of the love and fulfillment derived through relationships.

  - It is part of the healing process of pulling things in order and achieving closure in unresolved issues.

- **Gratitude:** Thankfulness or appreciation in acknowledgment of a benefit that one has received or will receive.

  - An attitude of gratitude nourishes the spirit and strengthens the ability to cope with different situations. During times of loss and crisis, clients or residents may benefit from a review of the positive aspects of their lives.

- **Transcendence:** The need to feel that there is greater reality beyond oneself, that one is connected to a greater power that surpasses common logical thinking, a source to draw on that empowers a person to achieve that which he or she cannot accomplish independently.

  - This affords clients life beyond material existence, and equips them to make sense of the difficulties they are experiencing.

- **Expression of Faith:** Religious beliefs and practices include prayers, worship, scripture reading, rituals, and celebrations.

  - Inability to express one's faith because of illness or disability leads to spiritual distress.

  - Clients may also at times feel resentful that God has seemingly abandoned them or is punishing them during periods of illness and suffering, which may lead to spiritual distress.

### *Supporting Spiritual Needs:*

Evidence-based practice suggests that strong spiritual beliefs foster health and healing. Therefore, it is therapeutically beneficial for CNAs to support clients' or residents' spirituality and assist them in fulfilling spiritual needs.

- Identifying needs: Asking about spiritual concerns during interactions promotes holistic care.

  - Check for visible cues. Depression, flat affect, crying, distressing statements and other observable signs could be considered red flags for spiritual distress, e.g. "Why did God allowed this to happen?"

- Offering self: Make yourself available to the client or resident. The rapport and trust that the client or resident feels toward the nurse assistant facilitates sharing of deep feelings.

  - CNAs need to honor this trust and be available for the exploration of feelings, not just by being physically present but fully present without being distracted.

- There may be moments when you don't know how to respond to a client's spiritual needs, especially if their beliefs differ from your own. In these situations, listen attentively and encourage communication.

- Honoring client's belief and practices: Expression of faith can be reflected in the client's or resident's rituals, diet, time and frequency of prayers, abstinence and celebration of certain occasions like the Sabbath or special feasts.

  - Acknowledge and respect the client's or resident's beliefs and practices non-judgmentally even if they differ from your own.

  - Never impose your own beliefs on a client.

  - Allow the client to express or exercise these practices to the extent allowed by policy.

- Providing client opportunities for solitude: Uninterrupted time or a moment of silence allows personal communication with one's God or other higher powers.

  - Allow and arrange schedules for the client or resident to have periods of solitude when he or she can offer prayers, reflect, meditate, reach out within himself or herself and listen for answers from their higher power.

- Praying with or for the client: Research evidence supports the positive relationship between prayer, health, and healing.

  - Prayers can be specific like that the therapy will alleviate the client's pain.

  - CNAs who are not comfortable offering prayers themselves can ask coworkers to pray with and for their clients who so desire.

- Promoting hope: When clients believe in the future and the possibility of positive outcomes or things to come, they are likely to commit to goals and actions, e.g. compliance to therapy and active involvement in one's care.

  - The potential of experiencing hopelessness and depression is very real, especially for clients and residents who are afflicted with serious illness and disabilities. Hopelessness interferes with self-care and healing, draining one's energies that are needed to combat life's challenges.

  - To promote hope, establish a trusting relationship with your client so he or she will be more comfortable in expressing feelings.

  - Facilitate client's practices, refer to clergy if appropriate.

- Guide client in a life review to highlight past successes in facing life's challenges.

- Use music and humor therapeutically.

- Alert: Client's faith can enable him or her to be comforted in believing that the current challenges serve a positive purpose for God.

## Spiritual Distress

Spiritual distress can result from declining health of the client or significant others, losses, awareness of mortality and even conflicts between beliefs and medical regimen. The client or resident may question his or her faith and beliefs.

### Checking for Signs of Spiritual Distress:

- Anger
- Anxiety
- Complaints
- Cynicism
- Crying
- Depression
- Expression of guilt
- Hopelessness
- Withdrawal or isolation
- Powerlessness
- Low self-esteem
- Suicidal thoughts
- Fatigue
- Poor appetite
- Sleep disturbance

### Pointers in Addressing Spiritual Distress:

- Help client or resident identify factors contributing to spiritual distress.

- Support client's or resident's spiritual practices. Provide or allow use of Bible/Koran, religious articles, inspirational music and periods of solitude. Read scriptures or arrange for someone to do so.

- Pray with or for the client or resident if this does not violate the client's or your own faith.

- Refer client or resident to clergy, healer, support group, or other spiritual resources aligned with client's faith. Contact client's church for visitation and link client with community ministry if the client or resident desires so. Do not insist if the client wishes otherwise.

- *Alert:* Do not challenge the client's or the resident's religious beliefs and values or attempt to change them.

## RELIGIOUS BELIEFS AND PRACTICES

Provided below are the highlights for several different religions to guide you in dealing with the clients with varied spiritual needs.

**Christianity:**

*Roman Catholic:*

- Express faith usually in formulated creeds or prayers, e.g. Apostle's Creed, Rosary.

- Fasting during Lent is common. They may refuse meat or meals during Holy Week.

- Priest provides communion, Sacrament of the Sick, and hears confession.

- Objects of spiritual expression include rosary beads, medallions, statues, Bible and novena references.

*Protestant:*

- **Seventh-Day Adventist:** Health lifestyle practices are promoted as the body is a temple of the Holy Spirit.

  - Prohibited: alcohol, tobacco, coffee, tea, recreational drugs, pork, shellfish, fish without scales and fins.

  - Most are vegetarian.

  - Sabbath is observed on Saturday. May refuse treatment at this time.

  - Clergy provides communion.

- Reading Bible is important.

- **Salvation Army:** Follow the Bible as the foundation or pillar of faith.

  - Scripture reading is emphasized.

  - Officers of a local Army can be requested for client visitation.

- **Pentecostal or Assemblies of God:** Believe in Jesus as the Savior.

  - Abstain from tobacco, alcohol, and illegal drugs.

  - Believe in divine healing through prayer and laying of hands.

  - Communion is provided by the clergy.

- **Baptist:** Scripture reading is emphasized as the Bible is the word of God.

  - Abstain from alcohol.

  - Communion is provided by the clergy.

- **Quaker:** Believe God is personal and real.

  - Any believer can achieve communion with Jesus Christ without the intercession of clergy or church rituals.

  - No special death ceremonies observed because of the belief that the present life is part of God's kingdom.

  - Abstain from alcohol.

  - May oppose or refuse medications.

- **Presbyterian:** Jesus Christ is the Savior.

  - Communion is provided by the clergy.

  - Clergy or elders can provide prayers for the dying.

- **Disciples of Christ or Christian Church:** Jesus Christ is the Savior.

  - Communion provided by the clergy is part of regular Sunday worship.

- Clergy and elders can be requested for spiritual support.

- **Church of the Brethren:** Clergy provides communion, anointing of the sick for physical healing and spiritual well-being.

- **Methodist:** Believe in Jesus Christ as the Savior.

  - Communion provided by the clergy.

  - During illness, anointing of the sick, reading Bible and prayers are important.

  - Encourage organ donation.

- **Anglican or Episcopal:** Jesus Christ is the Savior.

  - Fasting not required though some may abstain from meat on Fridays.

  - Communion is provided by the clergy.

  - Anointing of the sick may be offered but not required.

- **Church of the Nazarene:** Believe in divine healing but openly accept medical treatment.

  - Abstain from tobacco and alcohol.

  - Communion is provided by the clergy.

- **Lutheran:** Believe in Jesus Christ as the Savior.

  - Clergy provides communion, anointing of the sick and service of Commendation of the Dying.

- **Mennonite:** Emphasize simple and plain lifestyle.

  - Abstain from alcohol.

  - During illness and crisis, prayers and anointing with oil are essential.

  - May refuse medication.

  - Women may desire to wear head covering during hospitalization.

  - Communion is provided twice a year with washing of the feet as part of the ceremony.

*Eastern Orthodox*: Includes Greek, Serbian, Russian and other Orthodox churches.

- Holy Spirit proceeds from the Father, rather than Father and Son; therefore, do not acknowledge the Pope.

- Fast from meat and dairy products on Wednesdays and Fridays of the Lent including other holy days.

- Use a different calendar for religious celebrations.

- Fast during Lent and before communion.

- Last rites must be provided by an ordained priest.

*Christian Science*: Religion based on use of faith for healing.

- May refuse drugs, psychotherapy, hypnotism, vaccination and other regimen.

- Use Christian Science health care workers and may desire to actively participate in own care.

*Jehovah's Witnesses:*

- Blood transfusions not accepted.

- Discourage use of tobacco and alcohol.

*Church of Jesus Christ of Latter Day Saints or Mormons:*

- No professional clergy. A member of the church priesthood may provide communion, anointing of the sick and laying of hands.

- Abstain from alcohol and caffeine.

- A sacred undergarment may be worn and removed only during emergencies.

- May refuse medical treatments and resort to divine healing with laying of hands.

*Unitarian*: Highly liberal branch of Christianity. God is a single being rather than a Trinity.

- Believe individuals are responsible for their own health state.

- Encourage organ donation.

## Islam:

Islam is the second largest monotheistic religion in the world. It was founded by the Prophet Mohammad who was a human messenger of God or Allah. The Koran is the main scripture.

- Koran cannot be touched by anyone who is considered unclean.

- May pray five times a day facing Mecca.

- Abstinence from pork and alcohol. Haram diet is prohibited, Halal is allowed diet.

- Washing is required even for the sick during prayer time.

- Accept medical practices to the extent possible.

- Women are not allowed to sign consent or make decisions without the husband.

- Reproductive matters should be discussed with same gender.

- May wear *taviz*, a black string with words from Koran.

- Organ donation not allowed.

- Death and dying:

  - Family or any practicing Muslim can pray with dying client.

  - Most prefer family to wash and prepare the body of the deceased.

  - CNAs can care for the body by wearing gloves.

  - Autopsy prohibited unless legally required.

  - The body is covered with several white linens.

## Judaism:

Judaism is a monotheistic religion, with the **Torah** as its foundational text. Jews generally observe Sabbath from sundown Friday to night fall Saturday. The three branches are:

- **Observant or Orthodox:** Strictly adheres to the tradition.

  - Use the divinely inspired five books of Moses known as Torah.

- Kosher Diet:

    o No meat and dairy products at the same time.

    o Prohibited: pork, shellfish, meat not slaughtered according to Jewish law.

- Strict restrictions during Sabbath:

    o No riding in a car, smoking, handling money, using telephone or watching television.

    o Medical treatment may be postponed until after Sabbath.

- Shaving for men: do not use razor, blade should not come in contact with skin. Beard is considered a sign of piety.

- Men wear skullcaps at all times.

- Men will not touch any woman other than those in his family.

- Married women cover hair.

- Witness needs to be present when person prays for health so that if death occurs, family will be protected by God.

- If death occurs on Sabbath, Orthodox persons cannot handle the body but nurse aide or other staff can care for the body with gloves.

- Body must be buried within 24 hours; autopsy not allowed.

- Any removed body part must be returned for burial with the remaining body.

- **Conservative:** Observe same basic laws as Orthodox; may only cover heads during worship and prayer; autopsy may be permitted.

- **Reform:** Less stringent in adhering to laws.

    - Do not strictly follow Kosher diet.

    - Do not wear skullcaps.

    - Men can touch women.

    - Attend temples on Fridays but do not follow restriction during Sabbath.

### *Hinduism:*

Hinduism is the dominant religion, or way of life, of the Indian subcontinent with many diverse traditions. It is considered the world's oldest religion. There are no scriptures, fixed doctrines or common worship.

- Believe in karma and reincarnation. Every person is born into position based on the deeds in the previous life.

- Illness and disabilities maybe perceived as a sin or fault from the previous life.

- Most are vegetarian.

- Abstain from alcohol and tobacco.

### *Buddhism:*

Buddhism is a nontheistic religion or **dharma**, a "right way of living," that encompasses a variety of traditions, beliefs, and practices largely based on the **teachings** attributed to **Siddhartha Gautama**, commonly known as the Buddha, "the awakened one."

- Believe enlightenment is found in individual meditation rather than communal worship.

- Follow the moral code known as the Eightfold Path which leads to Nirvana, the highest form of liberation and enlightenment.

- Most are vegetarian.

- Abstain from alcohol and tobacco.

- May refuse medications and treatments, especially on holy days.

- Require private, uninterrupted periods of meditation.

# COMMUNICATION

## TERMS TO REMEMBER:

- **Attentive Listening:** Showing care for the needs or desires of others by paying close attention to the client during conversation.

- **Communication:** Any means of exchanging information or feelings between two or more people.

- **Genuineness:** Being true or authentic to one's message and character as conveyed in the care of a client.

- **Intimate Distance:** Ranges from touching to about 18 inches (46 cm) apart, and is reserved for lovers, children, close family members, friends, and pet animals.

- **Personal Space:** The region surrounding a person they regard as psychologically theirs.

- **Personal Distance:** Begins about an arm's length away; starting around 18 inches (46 cm) from the person and ending about 4 feet (122 cm) away. This space is used in conversations with friends, to chat with associates, and in group discussions.

- **Public Distance:** Includes anything more than 8 feet (2.4 m) away, and is used for speeches, lectures, and theater. Public distance is essentially that range reserved for larger audiences.

- **Social Distance:** Ranges from 4 to 8 feet (1.2 m - 2.4 m) away from the person and is reserved for strangers, newly formed groups, and new acquaintances.

- **Therapeutic Communication:** The face-to-face process of interacting that focuses on advancing the physical and emotional well-being of a patient.

## SKILLS TO MASTER:

- Understanding and using paralanguage

- Integrating cultural, religious, and personal attributes of clients in communication

- Active and attentive listening

- Identifying and eliminating communication barriers

- Mastering therapeutic phrases or statements

- Reading and interpreting clients nonverbal cues

- Self-management of emotions and expressions of feelings

- Using appropriate communication channels

- Assisting client with communication aids

Communication is from the Latin word *"communicare"* which means to establish a sense of commonness with others, to share information, signals, or messages in the form of ideas and feelings. It is a dynamic social process which involves the use of language, gestures, or symbols so that ideas are transmitted, received, and understood by the persons involved.

During interpersonal contacts with clients or residents, CNAs communicate with them about the tasks that are to be and are being performed as well as communicate with other members of the team for necessary care. In health care, communication is a dynamic process used to gather data, to teach and persuade, and to express caring and comfort. It is an integral part of the helping relationship.

**Developing Communication Skills**

CNAs who communicate effectively are better able to elicit information, initiate interventions, support change that promotes health, and prevent legal problems that may possibly arise in the provision of care. Strong communication processes are built on trusting relationships between the client and support persons. Following are some tips to enhance your communication skills while working as a certified nursing assistant:

- *Improve your observation skills.* As a CNA, you have to take initiative for creating cordial relationships with the client. Observe the client's or resident's behaviors. This will help you decide on the strategies of communication to be used in the relationship. Is the client irritable, restless, or in pain?

- *Establish rapport by introducing yourself and your role.* Give a brief introduction with your name, job title, and the responsibilities you have been assigned. A clear and to-the-point introduction will be helpful for the client to get easily acquainted to you. Show interest and positive regard with the use of a warm smile and genuine expressions.

- *Always greet your client with a warm and decent tone upon entering the room.* Ask them about their day, health, general mood, and related interests.

- *Before performing any task, explain the purpose of the procedure and how it will be carried out.* Allow the client to ask questions or express any doubts or concerns about the procedure. Encourage their active participation if warranted.

- *Attentive listening:* Pay full attention and convey interest in the client during interactions.

- *Effective reporting*: Reporting should be done in a concise, organized, timely, accurate, and clear manner.

- *Excellent language skills*: Be sensitive and wise in the use of words when conversing with the client. Choose those that deliver your message in a clear and therapeutic way.

## COMMUNICATION PROCESS

Face-to-face communication involves a sender, a message, a receiver, and a response or feedback. In its simplest form, communication is a two-way process involving the sending and receiving of a message. Because the intent of communication is to elicit a response, the process is ongoing or continuous wherein the receiver of the message then becomes the sender of the response and the original sender becomes the receiver.

- **Sender:** originator of information.

  - Source-encoder: the person or group sending the message must have an idea or reason for communicating (source) and must put the idea or feeling into a form that can be transmitted.

  - Encoding: selection of specific signs or symbols (codes) to transmit the message, e.g. the language and words to be used, arrangement of the words, and the choice of tone and gestures.

- **Message:** information being transmitted.

  - What is actually said or written, the body language that accompanies the words, and how the message is transmitted.

  - Channel: the medium used to convey the message, and it can target the different senses of the receiver.

  - Talking face-to-face with a person may be more effective in some instances than telephoning or writing a message.

- Written communication is often appropriate for long explanations or for communication that needs to be preserved. It can also be utilized for clients with hearing impairment or inability to produce words.

- Context: the setting of communication.

- **Receiver:** recipient of information.

  - This is the listener, who must listen, observe, and attend.

  - Decoder: the one who must perceive what the sender intended (interpretation).

  - Perception uses all of the senses to receive verbal and nonverbal messages.

  - To decode means to relate the message perceived to the receiver's storehouse of knowledge and experience and to sort out the meaning of the message.

  - If the meaning of the decoded message matches the intent of the sender, then the communication has been effective.

- **Feedback:** return response.

  - The response is the message the receiver returns to the sender.

  - It can be verbal, nonverbal, or both.

  - It also allows the sender to correct or reword a message.

*Themes of Communication:*

- **Content:** conversation may appear superficial but careful attention to the underlying theme helps the CNA identify problem areas while providing insight into the client's self-concept.

- **Mood:** emotion or affect that the client communicates to the nurse aide and others. It includes appearance, facial expressions, and gestures that reflect the client's feelings.

- **Interaction:** how the client reacts or interacts with the nurse assistant, including how the client relates and what role he or she assumes when communicating with the nurse and others.

*Modes of communication:*

- **Verbal:** written or spoken words.

- Largely conscious because people choose the words they use.

- The words used vary among individuals according to culture, socioeconomic background, age, and education. Countless possibilities exist for the ways ideas are exchanged.

- A wide variety of feelings can be conveyed when people talk.

- When choosing words to say or write, nurse assistants need to consider pace and intonation, simplicity, clarity and brevity, timing and relevance, adaptability, credibility, and humor.

  o Pace and Intonation: the manner of speech will modify the impact of the message.

    • The intonation can express enthusiasm, sadness, anger, or amusement.

    • The pace may indicate interest, anxiety, boredom, or fear.

  o Simplicity: the use of commonly understood words. Nurse aides need to learn to select appropriate, understandable terms based on the age, knowledge, culture, and education of the client. When in doubt, use layman's terms.

  o Clarity and Brevity: a message that is direct and simple will be more effective.

    • Clarity: saying precisely what is meant.

    • Brevity: using the fewest words possible.

    • An aspect of this is congruence, or consistency, where the CNA's behavior or nonverbal communication matches the spoken words.

    • To ensure clarity, speak slowly and enunciate clearly.

  o Timing and Relevance: maintaining sensitivity to the client's needs and concerns.

    • Allow the client to respond first to social talk or chat to develop rapport.

    • Let the client express feelings and concerns.

  o Adaptability: spoken messages need to be altered in accordance with behavioral cues from the client.

    • What the nurse assistant says and how it is said must be individualized and carefully considered.

    o Credibility: worthiness of belief, trustworthiness, and reliability.

- Nurse assistant can foster credibility by being consistent, dependable, and honest.

- There is a need to be knowledgeable about what is being discussed and to have accurate information.

- Nurse assistants should convey confidence and certainty in what they are saying, while being able to acknowledge their limitations.

    o Humor: the physical act of laughter can be an emotional and physical release, reducing tension by providing a different perspective and promoting a sense of well-being.

- It is important to consider the client's perception of what is humorous, including the proper timing.

- While humor and laughter can help reduce stress and anxiety in the early and recovery stages of a crisis, it may be considered offensive or distracting at the peak of the crisis.

- **Nonverbal:** body movements (kinetics), space (proxemics), paralanguage (voice quality, way of message delivery), touch, and silence.

  - It is sometimes called body language.

  - Nonverbal communication often tells others more about what a person is feeling than what is actually said, because nonverbal behavior is controlled less consciously than verbal behavior.

  - It either reinforces or contradicts what is said verbally.

  - To observe nonverbal behavior efficiently requires a systematic assessment of the person's overall physical appearance, posture, gait, facial expressions, and gestures.

  - Whatever is observed, the nurse assistant needs to exercise caution in interpretation, always clarifying any observation with the client.

        o Personal Appearance: clothing and adornments can be sources of information about a person.

    - This may convey social and financial status, culture, religion, group association, and self-concept.

    - How a person dresses is often an indicator of how the person feels. Someone who is tired or ill may not have the energy or the desire to maintain their normal grooming. When a person who is known for grooming becomes lax about appearance, it may indicate loss of self-esteem or a physical illness.

o Posture and Gait: the ways people walk and carry themselves are often reliable indicators of self-concept, current mood, and health.

- Erect posture and an active, purposeful stride suggest a feeling of well-being.

- Slouched posture and a slow, shuffling gait suggest depression or physical discomfort.

- Tense posture and a rapid, determined gait suggest anxiety or anger.

- The posture of people when sitting or lying can also indicate feelings or mood.

- The nurse assistant should clarify the meaning of the observed behavior by describing to the client what he or she sees and then asking what it means.

o Facial expression: feelings of surprise, fear, anger, disgust, happiness and sadness can be conveyed by facial expressions, as this is the most expressive part of the body.

- Although the face may express the person's genuine emotions, it can also be controlled and may not reflect what the person is really feeling.

- Nurse assistants need to be aware of their own expressions and what they are communicating to others. Clients are quick to notice the health care member's facial expression, particularly when the client feels unsure or uncomfortable.

- It is impossible to control all facial expressions, but the nurse assistant must learn to control expressions of feelings such as fear of disgust in some circumstances.

- Eye contact is also an essential element of facial communication. Mutual eye contact acknowledges recognition of the other person and a willingness to maintain communication.

o Gestures: hand and body gestures may emphasize and clarify the spoken words, or they may occur without words to indicate a particular feeling or to give a sign.

- For people with special communication problems, such as the deaf, the hands are invaluable in communication with the use of sign language.

**Criteria for Successful Communication:**

- *Feedback:* the return response.

- *Appropriateness*: the response directly answers the question.

- *Efficiency*: the language used is understood by the communicators.

- *Flexibility*: the absence of under control and over control known as communication balance.

## THERAPEUTIC COMMUNICATION

Therapeutic communication promotes understanding and can help establish a constructive relationship between the nurse assistant and the client. It is client- and goal-directed. It is important to understand how the client views the situation and feels about it before responding.

*Characteristics of Therapeutic Communication:*

- **Clear:** it contains words that can be understood; allows for response from the client; deals with cognitive and emotional aspects of the client.

- **Consistent:** implies the same message through time.

- **Direct:** contains the essential points that need to be communicated.

*Techniques of Communication*

| Communication Technique | Sample statement |
|---|---|
| Accepting | "I acknowledge what you said…" |
| Clarifying | "What do you mean by…?" |
| Exploring | "Tell me more about it." |
| Focusing | " Kindly tell me to whom are you referring to…?" |
| Giving broad opening | "What are your thoughts today?" |
| Giving information | "The reason for my being here is…" |
| Giving recognition | "I notice you've washed your face…" |
| Offering one's self | "I'll stay with you for awhile." |
| Offering general leads | "Tell me about that…" |
| Observing | "I notice that you're biting your nails." |
| Placing the event in time or sequence | "When did this happen?" |

| Presenting reality | "I understand that hearing a voice is real to you, but I don't hear it." |
|---|---|
| Restating | Client: "I stayed awake all night." <br><br> CNA: "Are you saying you have difficulty sleeping?" |
| Reflecting | Client: "I can't imagine that my spouse can do this to me." <br><br> CNA: "This causes you to feel angry." |
| Suggesting collaboration | "We can talk about how you are coping with your anxiety…" |
| Summarizing | "In the past hour, you and I have talked about…" |
| Using silence | (just stay physically available to the client) |
| Validating | "Tell me whether my interpretation of what I thought you said is what you really mean." |

*Pointers in communication techniques:*

- Paralanguage includes the quality of the voice and the way the message is delivered.

- Listening requires careful concentration to guide the conversation to a specific goal.

- The use of silence during interaction also indicates that the CNA is listening.

- Events that curtail communication can produce emotional disturbance.

- To encourage a non-communicative client to talk, the nurse assistant should focus on non-threatening subjects.

## BARRIERS TO COMMUNICATION

Nurse assistants need to recognize barriers or non-therapeutic responses to effective communication. Failure to listen, improperly decoding the client's intended message, and placing the nurse aide's needs above the client's needs are major barriers.

| Communication Barrier | Sample statement |
|---|---|
| Stereotyping | "Men don't cry" <br><br> "Women are complainers." |

| Agreeing and disagreeing | Client: "I don't think Dr. X is very good."<br><br>CNA: "Dr. X is the head of the department and is a very good and excellent doctor." |
| --- | --- |
| Being defensive | Client: "Those night nurses are just sitting around and talking all night. They didn't even answer my call immediately."<br><br>CNA: "The entire team literally runs around all night. You're not the only patient you know." |
| Challenging | Client: "I feel as if I am dying."<br><br>CNA: "How can you feel that way when your pulse is 60?" |
| Probing | Client: "I didn't ask the doctor when he was here."<br><br>CNA: "Why didn't you?" |
| Testing | "Who do you think you are?"<br><br>"Do you think I am not busy?" |
| Rejecting | "I don't want to discuss that. Let's talk about…"<br><br>"I can't talk to you now. I'm going for lunch break." |
| Changing topics and subjects | Client: "I'm separated from my wife. Do you think it's time to find a new partner?"<br><br>CNA: "I see that you are 40-years old and you like gardening. I have a beautiful rose garden. If you want, I can walk you to the park nearby to also see the garden there." |
| Unwarranted reassurance | "You'll feel better soon."<br><br>"Don't worry. You will be okay." |
| Passing judgment | "What you did was wrong."<br><br>"That's not good enough." |
| Giving common advice | Client: "Should I move from my home to a nursing home?"<br><br>CNA: "If I were you, I'd go to a nursing home where you will have good meals and rest." |

**Communication with Elders:**

Older adults may have physical or cognitive problems that necessitate nursing interventions for improvement of communication skills. Actions directed toward improvement of communication in elderly clients are as follows:

- Make sure assistive devices, glasses, and hearing aids are being used and are in good working order.

- Make referrals as necessary.

- Use communication aids like boards and pictures.

- Minimize environmental distractions.

- Speak in short, simple sentences, one subject at a time. Repeat or reinforce what is said when necessary.

- Always face the person when speaking.

- Include family and friends in the conversation.

- Use reminiscing to maintain memory connections and to enhance self-identity and self-esteem in the elderly.

- Find out what has been important and has meaning to the elderly client and try to maintain these things as much as possible.

## COMMUNICATION AMONG HEALTH PROFESSIONALS

Effective communication among health professionals is as important as the promotion of therapeutic communication with clients to provide quality and continuity of care. Those health care workers who are confident in their communication abilities to discuss their concerns with their co-workers are more satisfied and committed to staying in health care.

Standard for skilled communication:

CNAs must be as proficient in communication skills as they are in clinical skills.

- Focus on finding solutions and achieving desirable outcomes.

- Seek to protect and advance collaborative relationships among colleagues.

- Invite and hear relevant perspectives from other members of the team.

- Observe goodwill and mutual respect to build consensus and arrive at common understanding.

- Demonstrate congruence between words and actions.

- Learn how to use communication technologies in the facility.

# CLIENT'S RIGHTS

## TERMS TO REMEMBER:

- **Confidentiality**: A set of rules that limits access or places restrictions on certain types of information from patient communication.

- **Dignity**: An individual or group's sense of self-respect and self-worth, physical and psychological integrity, and empowerment.

- **Elder Abuse**: Harm to older adults by trusted individuals in a manner that causes pain or distress.

- **Elderspeak**: A specialized speech style used by younger adults when addressing older adults. The speaker makes accommodations that include producing shorter, less complex sentences, using simpler vocabulary, filler words, fragmented sentences, lexical filters, and repetition.

- **Neglect**: A condition that occurs when the health care worker fails to provide minimal physical and emotional care to his or her client.

- **Privacy**: Physical and personal space, clothing, and other measures to ensure freedom from physical interference.

- **Patient Rights**: Legal and ethical issues in the provider-patient relationship, including a person's right to privacy, the right to quality medical care without prejudice, the right to make informed decisions about care and treatment options, and the right to refuse treatment.

- **Respect**: Esteem for a person's sense of worth.

## SKILLS TO MASTER:

- Educating self and others on Patient's Rights

- Providing competent clinical skills

- Accurate documentation

- Prompt reporting of client's concerns

- Collaboration with the team and patient ombudsman

- Identifying signs of patient abuse and neglect

- Reporting abuse cases to legal authorities

- Communication skills

- Good customer service skills

Formalized in 1948, the Universal Declaration of Human Rights recognizes "the inherent dignity" and the "equal and unalienable rights of all members of the human family." It is on the basis of this concept and the fundamental dignity and equality of all human beings that the notion of client or patient rights was developed.

The Universal Declaration of Human Rights has been instrumental in enshrining the notion of human dignity in international law, providing a legal and moral grounding for improved standards of care on the basis of our basic responsibilities towards each other as members of the "human family," and giving important guidance on critical social, legal, and ethical issues.

There exist variations in local and state legislation and administration of patients' rights. CNAs must keep in mind that it is important for clients or patients to receive treatment consistent with the dignity and respect they are owed as human beings. This means providing, at minimum, equitable access to quality medical care, ensuring patients' privacy and the confidentiality of their medical information, informing patients and obtaining their consent before employing a medical intervention, and providing a safe clinical environment.

## RIGHTS OF RESIDENTS OR PATIENTS

Clients or patients and residents must be given a copy of their special rights when they come to a hospital, assisted living facility, or nursing home. As advocates, nurse assistants can also help reinforce education of clients about their rights in the health care setting.

All patients and residents have a right to:

- Respect and dignity

- Privacy and confidentiality

- Freedom from abuse and neglect

- Control their own money or resources

- Have their personal property

- Know about their medical condition and treatments

- Choose their own doctor(s)

- Make decisions about their medical care

- Receive competent care

- Practice religious and social freedom

- Receive accurate bills for services given

- Complain and be heard

## RESPECT & DIGNITY

Among the most important human needs is the desire for respect and dignity. That need doesn't change when a person becomes ill or disabled. Indeed, it may grow even stronger. We must:

- Speak to clients with respect. Conversing with your clients should convey a kind, helpful, and polite attitude.

- Utilize good communication skills.

- When talking to clients or residents, call them by their name. Include a title according to the client's preference. Avoid addressing them with 'momma', 'poppa', 'sweetie' or 'honey' as these are unprofessional.

- Encourage the client to express feelings and concerns. Give them enough time to talk with you. Do NOT look like you are in a hurry. Listen attentively with interest.

- Avoid Elderspeak. NEVER treat an adult like a child. Do NOT talk 'baby talk' to adults. Elderspeak speech style is often patronizing in nature and resembles baby talk, which refers to how adults address babies and young children. It results from stereotypes about the cognitive abilities of older persons.

- Assist clients and residents so they can be as independent as they can. Help them with their self-care and activities of daily living.

- Promote personal care and grooming to enhance self-worth or sense of well-being. You must make them look clean, shaved, and without dirty fingernails.

- Attend to the client's or resident's needs immediately. Do not allow him or her to be soaked in urine or excreta, or go through the day dirty or with a bad odor. These things can rob a person's dignity.

- Provide clients or residents with as many choices or alternatives as possible. Promote a sense of independence or self-reliance in decision-making unless their choice can cause them harm or can harm others. For example, let the client choose his own clothes for the activity.

- Provide client or resident privacy. Keep him or her draped covered when providing physical care. Pull the curtains around the bed. Close the door when you help him dress or use the bathroom.

- Make the client or resident feel unique and special each and every time you are with them.

## PRIVACY AND CONFIDENTIALITY

Quality patient care requires the communication of relevant information between health professionals and/or health systems. Nurse assistants and other health professionals who regularly work with patients and their confidential medical records should contribute to the development of standards, policies, and laws that protect patient privacy and the confidentiality of health records and information.

Protection of privacy/confidentiality is essential to the trusting relationship between health care providers and patients. Clients or residents do not lose their right to privacy because they are in a hospital or nursing home. They also do not lose this right when they have home health care.

- Allow client or resident to talk privately with family, friends, and other patients or residents. Do not interfere or eavesdrop. Give people a private place to talk with ease.

- Clients or residents have the right to keep their personal things in the area. Do not attempt to open a patient's closet or pocketbook without getting their permission. When attending to a client in his or her home, ask the client's permission first before entering any area or using any articles.

- Knock on the client's or resident's door before entering. The client's room is considered their personal or private space.

- Provide personal privacy when bathing or caring for a patient.

- Health care workers, including nursing assistants, should NEVER tell a person's diagnosis or condition to anyone who is NOT caring for the patient. Don't discuss confidential information with other people, even family members, without the patient's permission.

- Secure client's or resident's records in a safe place to be accessed only by members of the team caring for him or her.

- Do not disclose any information about the client or resident to other clients or to unknown people who have called the station.

## FREEDOM FROM ABUSE & NEGLECT

Abuse and neglect have different meanings, but are both associated with the emotional and physical well-being of a person. Abuse means maltreatment of a person, either physically or psychologically, and neglect means the failure to give proper care to a person, either physically or psychologically.

Abuse is the misuse of power and trust, whereas neglect is the deliberate act of forgetting and not caring. Abusing is harming someone or something, whereas neglect is not preventing the harmful action.

Many elders, children, women, and young adults with physical or mental deficits are at risk for abuse and neglect especially when they become highly dependent on others to meet their needs. Abuse and neglect in health care settings is a tragic reality facing many families.

Unfortunately, in health care settings like nursing homes, neglect and abuse can be a "hidden problem" because the victims are often not capable of expressing pain or reporting the neglect or abuse on their own. Thus, it is extraordinarily important that nursing assistants be watchful for any signs or symptoms of abuse. Any one or more of the following signs could be evidence of nursing home abuse or neglect and warrants investigation:

- Bedsores or decubitus ulcers

- Skin rashes, lesions, tears

- Standing urine and/or feces odor

- Lack of attention to resident's personal hygiene

- Falls resulting from lack of adequate precautions or assistance

- Bruises, contusions

- Fractures

- Significant weight loss

- Dehydration

- Disorientation

- Depression or isolation

- Unexplained mood changes

- Fear or anxiety

- Unexplained refusal or inability to communicate

- Presence of unjustified chemical or physical restraints

*Abuse* can come in many forms, such as: physical or verbal maltreatment, injury, assault, violation, rape, unjust practices, crimes, or other *types* of aggression. The most common forms of abuse confronting members of the health care team are physical, emotional or mental, sexual, or financial.

- *Physical abuse.* Physical abuse involves the use of a physical force, e.g. a punch, slap, push, or pinch. Elders are often physically abused with rough treatment, especially those with cognitive impairments like dementia. Grabbing a client forcefully out of bed is physical abuse. Check for signs of physical abuse like skin tears, bruises and fractures, or bone dislocations.

- *Mental abuse.* This causes the person to have mental pain or psychological trauma, e.g. yelling and obscene name calling. Dealing with an elderly resident by treating her like a child, locking her in the room or withdrawing privileges are forms of psychological abuse. Signs of mental abuse are fear, crying, sadness, withdrawal, and sleep disturbances. Emotional abuse is inadequate emotional or physical care, or isolation.

- *Sexual abuse.* Sexual abuse is sexual contact of any kind without the consent of the other person. It includes forced or unwanted sexual contact and harassment, e.g. touching, fondling, and rape.

- *Financial abuse.* Financial abuse is the improper or illegal use of the victim's money. It means to steal, withhold money, or prevent access to financial accounts.

Neglect does NOT involve an act that is wrong. Neglect is NOT doing something that should be done. Men, women, and people of all ages can be neglected. Neglect has also many types, such as physical, educational, medical, and emotional neglect.

- *Physical neglect*. Physical neglect is the failure or delay in providing healthcare, abandonment, and expulsion. Neglect also includes leaving a child under inadequate supervision, nutrition, hygiene, and clothing, which may endanger their safety and welfare.

- *Mental neglect* or psychological neglect. Delaying or refusing to provide physiological care to a person, and allowing abusive behaviors.

- *Financial neglect*. If any elderly person lives in the home with a daughter and the daughter does not take care of the bills or spends the elderly person's money on things not directly related to that person, then this is financial neglect.

## CONTROL OVER FINANCIAL RESOURCES

Clients and residents who are able to make decisions can, and should, have control of their finances. They should be allowed to decide and plan how to spend their money whether the expenses are related to their health care or not. In the event that the client or resident is no longer able to make decisions on his or her own, legal arrangements can be made for another person or significant other to decide on his or her behalf.

Clients should also be informed of the financial aspect or costs of his or her care, not only from the beginning of the management, but also with regular updates. This will allow them to prepare for the necessary expenses such as diagnostic tests, medical or surgical therapies, and other related health care services. Options or alternatives should be discussed with the clients and their support system to better plan for their care.

For clients or residents with financial difficulties, they can be referred to social services or agencies that can help them cover the costs of the health care services needed. They also have the right to be properly educated on their medical insurance regarding the coverage and means of fund disbursement during their therapies or hospital stay.

## RIGHT TO INFORMATION

A patient's right to know encompasses various types of disclosure regarding health care. It typically covers health care outcomes, physician profiles, malpractice reporting, hospital performance, and safety information. The term may be used in a broader sense to include a patient's right to know their medical condition, unanticipated outcomes, risks, etc.

- Clients or residents have the right to accurate and easy-to-understand information about their health plan, health care professionals, and health care facilities.

- Clients and residents must know about:

- their condition

- the benefits and risks of a treatment before agree to it

- alternative treatment options

- If they speak another language, have a physical or mental disability, or just don't understand something, help should be given to enable them to make informed health care decisions.

- They must be told how their medicines and treatments can help them, including possible side effects or potential harm.

- Nursing assistants may be asked to give information to a patient or resident. Talk to the client or resident in simple words they can understand.

- If the client asks you a question that you cannot answer, report this question to the nurse.

- The clients must also be made aware of their patient rights and responsibilities in the hospital, nursing home, or health care facility.

## RIGHT TO REFUSE TREATMENT

Every competent adult has the right to refuse unwanted medical treatment. This is part of the right of every individual to choose what will be done to his or her own body, and it applies even when refusing treatment means that the person may die. The right to refuse treatment hinges on that person being of sound mind and being able to decide for themselves. In many cases, a patient might not be able to make that call.

- A person might decide against having a recommended treatment for any number of reasons.

  - For religious reasons, some patients do not want to receive blood transfusions.

  - The treatment is too risky or expensive, or even if the treatment works, there is little or no chance it will get them back to a quality of life they could enjoy or accept.

  - Many do not want life-sustaining treatments like ventilators or feeding tubes if these treatments are only going to prolong the dying process.

- Having the right to refuse medical treatment does not mean that a decision to forgo treatment will be accepted without question at all times.

  - Any time a patient turns down a recommended treatment, it means that he or she and the health care team view the situation differently.

- It is the client's job is to consider all the options and decide what is best *for him or her.*

  - What is most important from the medical point of view may not be most important from the patient's point of view, because goals and values may differ.

- As long as the client has been given all the relevant information about his or her treatment options and knows the risks and benefits of each option, including the risks and benefits of turning down treatment, the client's wishes come first.

## RELIGIOUS AND SOCIAL FREEDOM

All clients or residents have the right to freedom of religion and cultural expression. Nurse assistants ought to explore, understand, and acknowledge the cultural and religious preferences of their clients.

- Acknowledge and allow religious and cultural practices unless contraindicated to the client's welfare and safety of the institution.

- Religious activities should never be forced upon a client, especially if these are not aligned with their beliefs and practices.

- Help clients go to the religious groups they choose.

- Encourage them to choose the groups and activities that they want.

- Help them get to any social, recreational, and/or patient rights groups that they want to attend.

## ACCURATE BILLS

Laws state that all patients and residents have a right to a bill that ONLY reflects those supplies or services they actually availed. The billing statement or the breakdown of costs and expenses should also be clear and properly explained to the concerned party.

In as much as nursing assistants are not directly involved in billing, upholding the client's right to information about his or her bills may include:

- Not charging a supply, such as a urinary drainage bag, dressings, or any other articles that the client didn't use or avail.

- Referring the client to the charge nurse if he or she wants to speak to someone about their bill for clarification.

## RIGHT TO COMPLAIN

All health care facilities have a client or patient ombudsman. A patient ombudsman informs the clients or patients of their rights and assists them as necessary in submitting an objection or complaint concerning treatment, or a claim for indemnity for professional negligence.

- Clients who are dissatisfied with their care or treatment can be assisted to properly make an objection to the director of the health care unit.

- The idea of submitting a complaint or objection is to provide clients with a straightforward and flexible way of passing their opinion to the health care unit.

- The formal complaint or objection allows the health care units the opportunity to rectify or address the situation without delay.

- When the complaint involves liability for patient injury, indemnification liability, or disciplinary proceedings, the client's or patient's ombudsman will assist the client in initiating the matter and submitting it to the appropriate department or will further provide guidance in the proceedings of the complaint.

- As a nurse assistant, notify the charge nurse if the client or resident has a complaint or concern. The nurse will then attend to the client and refer to the patient ombudsman if warranted.

- The best management of complaints is still prevention. Most complaints or objections can be avoided with the provision of competent care and a good customer service approach.

- Never argue with the client or act defensively toward the client's complaints. These should be dealt with professionally.

# LEGAL AND ETHICAL BEHAVIOR

## TERMS TO REMEMBER:

- **Accountability**: Answerability, blameworthiness, and liability in one's own decisions and actions.

- **Ethics**: A system of moral principles or moral standards governing conduct.

- **Ethical Codes**: Systematic guidelines for shaping ethical behavior that answer the normative questions of what beliefs or values should be morally accepted.

- **Ethical Responsibilities:** The specific values expected of a CNA.

- **Ethical Problems**: Situations where there are conflicts between one or more values and uncertainty about the correct course of action.

- **Ethical or Moral Uncertainty**: When a nurse feels indecision or a lack of clarity, or is unable to even know what the moral problem is, while at the same time feeling uneasy or uncomfortable.

- **Ethical Distress**: Situations where nursing assistants know or believe they know the right thing to do, but for various reasons (including fear or circumstances beyond their control) do not or cannot take the right action to prevent a particular harm.

- **Ethical or Moral Disengagement**: Disregard for normal ethical commitments. A CNA may become apathetic or disengage to the point of being unkind, uncompassionate, or even cruel to clients or other health care workers.

- **Ethical Violations**: Actions or failures to act that breach fundamental duties to clients or to colleagues and other health care providers.

- **Malpractice:** Professional misconduct or any unreasonable lack of skill or fidelity in the performance of professional duties.

- **Negligence:** An action which a reasonably prudent nursing assistant would have not done, or the failure to do an action which a reasonably prudent nursing assistant would have done, under similar circumstances.

## SKILLS TO MASTER

- Documentation and reporting

- Following chain of command

- Identifying and understanding client's or resident's rights

- Knowing the different laws and policies affecting the CNA practice and applying these in the performance of duties

- Communication with clients, their significant others, and members of the health care team

- Practicing privacy and confidentiality in rendering care

- Addressing client's or resident's complaints or grievances and reporting these to the supervisor and coordinating with the patient ombudsman

- Identifying and reporting cases of abuse and other clients' rights violations

- Exercising necessary precautions in performing physical care and maintaining environmental safety

As a professional member of the health care team, there are certain ethical and legal issues that must be upheld by Certified Nurse Assistants. Nurse assistants make decisions every day that must take into account laws and ethical standards. Therefore, in order to make appropriate decisions, nurse assistants require an understanding of how laws, ethics, and health care interface. An ethical issue can occur in any health care situation where profound moral questions of "rightness" or "wrongness" underlie professional decision-making and the beneficent care of clients or residents.

Professionalism reflects how one behaves when at work. It includes grooming, how one dresses, the choice of words, and the things one shares with others. For a nursing assistant, professionalism means following the care plan, being careful in making client observations, and always reporting and documenting accurately.

*Pointers in Professionalism:*

Part of professionalism and legal responsibilities involves following policies and procedures. Maintaining a professional and ethical relationship reduces the likelihood of liabilities and promotes quality care to the clients or residents. A CNA must keep in mind that his or her professional relationship with the client or resident encompasses the following:

- Keeping a positive professional attitude.

- Performing only the tasks assigned within the job description and the ones he or she is trained to do.

- Speaking politely and cheerfully to the client or resident regardless of personal mood.

- Never discussing your personal problems with the client or resident.

- Calling the client or resident by the name he or she prefers.

- Listening attentively to the client or resident.

- Always finding time to explain the procedural care before performing it.

- Following care practice protocols like hand washing and precautions to protect self and the clients.

*Professional Relationship with the Employer or Facility:*

As an employee in contract with a facility, the nursing assistant also must maintain a professional relationship with his or her employer. That means:

- Maintaining a proactive attitude.

- Completing duties efficiently.

- Consistently following all policies and procedures.

- Always documenting and reporting carefully and correctly.

- Communicating problems with the appropriate members of the health care team.

- Reporting any concerns that prevent you from completing duties.

- Asking questions or clarifications on matters you don't understand or know.

- Taking directions or criticism without getting upset and learning from these to improve performance.

- Being clean and neatly dressed and groomed.

- Maintaining punctuality at work.

- Notifying employer if unable to work or perform duties.

- Respecting and following the chain of command.

- Participating in any education programs offered to advance your competence and to keep abreast of the health care policies.

- Being a positive role model in the facility.

*CNA Professional Qualities:*

To keep one's job as a CNA while contributing to the well-being of the clients or residents, a professional and ethical nursing assistant has to develop or cultivate the following qualities:

- **Compassionate:** caring, concerned, empathetic and understanding.

- **Honest:** observing fidelity or truthfulness.

- **Conscientious:** always doing one's best in the tasks assigned.

- **Dependable:** offering to meet client or resident needs and helping colleagues when needed.

- **Respectful:** showing positive regard toward clients or residents including their belongings and privacy.

- **Considerate:** being understanding of the client's or resident's feelings and concerns.

- **Unprejudiced:** treating all residents or clients the same regardless of their backgrounds.

- **Nonjudgmental:** acknowledging and accepting the clients or residents and their behaviors without judging or imposing one's opinions or standards.

Ethics and laws guide human behaviors. They protect clients' rights in receiving care and guide health care professionals in rendering services. **Ethics** is a branch of **philosophy** that involves systematizing, defending, and recommending concepts of right and wrong **conduct**.

The nursing assistants' legal and ethical behaviors include the following examples:

- Observing honesty or fidelity.

- Protecting client's or resident's privacy including the confidentiality of the case.

- Never becoming personally involved.

- Reporting actual or suspected cases of abuse of a client or resident and/or assisting the client or resident in reporting the case.

- Not performing unassigned tasks or functions beyond the scope of CNA practice.

- Reporting all client or resident observations and incidents.

- Documenting accurately in a timely manner.

- Following standard precautions and protocols.

Clients' or residents' rights pertain to the proper expected treatment and quality of service they ought to receive while in a health care facility. These rights serve as the guide in the ethical code of conduct of health care workers as well as a foundation in health care related policies and mandates.

**Omnibus Budget and Reconciliation Act (*OBRA*) of 1987**

OBRA 87 requires the health care facility to provide each client or resident with care that will enable the client "to attain or maintain the highest practicable physical, mental, and psychosocial well-being."

It requires the nursing home and the health care team to continuously evaluate the client's or resident's abilities to self-care and to communicate needs. The client or resident should be fully evaluated before admission and every year thereafter in regards to health, memory, activities, etc. The nursing home must develop plans to prevent the deterioration of a client's or resident's condition and further advance his or her interest. This federal mandate also sets minimum standards for Nursing Assistant Training to ensure the quality of care of patients or residents. As a client rights advocate, the nurse aide helps the client or resident to practice autonomy in his or her activities, schedules, and health care decisions.

This law identified the following rights of clients or residents:

- **Quality of life**: Residents have the right to the best care available. Dignity, choices, and self-autonomy are integral parts of this.

- **Services and activities to maintain high-level of wellness:** Residents must be given the necessary care to promote and maintain their well-being, allowing them to attain their optimum level of functioning.

- **Be fully informed regarding rights and services**: Residents must be made aware of the available care and services in the facility. They should also be educated about their legal rights and responsibilities while in the facility.

- **Participate in their own care:** Respect the residents' right to self-determination to decide what is best for them. They also have the right to refuse medication, treatment, or restraints, and choose their doctors or health care providers. Any changes in their conditions and management have to be coordinated with them.

- **Make independent choices:** Residents are allowed to make choices about the care and treatments they receive including personal concerns like what to wear and how to spend their time and resources.

- **Privacy and confidentiality**: Residents expect privacy with the different procedural care given to them. All information about them, e.g. medical conditions, test results, prognosis, and personal concerns disclosed are part of privileged communication which should be kept confidential and shared only to other members of the health care team.

- **Dignity, respect and freedom**: Residents must be dealt with respectfully, with positive regard, without any coercion, neglect, or any form of abuse.

- **Security of possessions**: Residents' personal belongings must be kept safe while in the health care setting. These should not be used, taken, or shared with anyone without prior permission from the owner.

- **Choices regarding transfers and discharges:** Any needed relocation or transfer from one area to another within or outside the facility must be coordinated first with the residents.

- **Voice complaints**: Residents have the right to complain without fear of punishment, without threat, and without their privileges and care being withheld in the process. The facility and health care workers must work to try to resolve these complaints if warranted.

- **Visitations from physician and family**: Residents have the right to receive visits from their doctors, friends, or significant others to meet their physical and psychosocial needs.

As nursing assistants mandated to follow the OBRA law, you can help protect the residents' rights and deal with them professionally and ethically with the following:

- Watch for and report violations of the residents' rights.

- Actively participate in the decision making of the residents in planning their care.

- Always clarify your role and explain the procedures before performing them.

- Never abuse a resident in any form: physically, emotionally, verbally, or sexually.

- Respect a resident's refusal of care or regimen and help him or her understand the consequences of the decision. Report the refusal to the nurse in charge immediately.

- Inform the charge nurse of the client's or resident's complaints or questions about the goals of care in the nursing care plan.

- Document accurately and truthfully.

- Never talk or gossip about a resident. This not only violates confidentiality but may also result in defamation or slander liability.

- Never enter a resident's room without knocking and asking permission.

- Do not accept personal gifts or money from the resident.

- Never open a resident's mail, luggage, or look through his or her belongings. Respect the resident's possessions.

- Promptly report observations regarding a resident's condition or care.

- Assist the resident in resolving any disputes and coordinate this with your supervisor.

## LEGAL LIABILITIES

### Abuse

Abuse means purposely causing physical, mental, or emotional pain or injury to the resident or client. Examples include:

- Forcefully shaving a resident

- Purposely embarrassing a resident

### Neglect

Neglect refers to the failure to provide needed care, e.g. deliberately ignoring a client or resident.

### Domestic Violence

This is abuse perpetrated by the spouse, children, or members of the family or household. This includes cases of child abuse, battered women, elderly abuse, spousal abuse, and rape.

### Workplace Violence

This refers to abuse by an employer or resident. It comes in varied forms like physical, verbal or sexual.

### Negligence

Negligence means the failure to provide the proper care for a resident that results in injury or harm.

- The nurse assistant failed to check that the resident's dentures were broken leading to oral injury with continuous use and feeding.

- The nurse assistant forgot to raise the side rails after morning care. The resident fell, sustaining a head injury.

### Breach of Confidentiality

As a nursing assistant, you may learn about a resident's state of health, finances, and personal and family relationships. You are legally and ethically obliged to keep all information confidential. Disclosing information would only be warranted with the resident's permission, and only then with the members of the health care team and for public safety. A breach in confidentiality means breaking the client's trust in you or the team.

### Invasion of Privacy

This legal term means violation of the resident's right to privacy by exposing his or her private affairs, body, name, or even photograph in public without the person's consent.

### Sexual Harassment

Sexual harassment occurs when one person requests or otherwise requires any sexual favor from another person, regardless of whether such demand, request, or requirement for submission is accepted.

### False Imprisonment

This is restraining of a client or resident in a bounded area without justification or consent. False imprisonment is a common-law felony and a tort punishable under both criminal and civil laws.

- It may arise when the nurse assistant locks a client or resident within a room or in a closet.

### Assault and Battery

This is the combination of two violent crimes: assault (the threat of violence) and battery (physical violence). This legal distinction exists only in jurisdictions that distinguish assault as *threatened* violence rather than *actual* violence.

- Alert: Performing procedural care to a client without his or her consent or against his or her will constitutes battery.

- Threatening a client with physical punishment like placing him or her in restraints or giving shots is a form of assault.

### Defamation

This act pertains to character assassination whether in the form of slander (oral or verbal. e.g. gossips) or libel (written).

## CLIENT'S OR RESIDENT'S MEDICAL RECORD

Careful charting is important for the following reasons:

- It is a means to guarantee clear and complete communication between the members of the health care team.

- Documentation is a legal record of all aspects of the resident's treatment. Medical records or charts can be used as legal evidence in court by virtue of subpoena duces tecum.

- Documentation is a double-edged sword. It protects both the client and the members of the health care team and the employer from liabilities.

- Documentation on the resident's record provides an up-to date record of their health status and care.

- Documentation promotes effective communication among the members of the team and continuity of client care.

### Guidelines in Documentation:

- Write notes immediately after the care is given.

- Notes should also follow chronological order according to the care performed.

- Write facts, not opinions or assumptions.

- Write as neatly as you can. Use black ink.

- If you make a mistake, draw a single line through the entry and write the correct word or phrase. Write error or mistaken entry above the crossed out word or words. Affix your signature, initials, and the date. Erasures and correction fluid are not allowed.

- Sign your full name and title with the correct date.

- Document as specified in the care plan or per facility policy. Some facilities have a "check-off" sheet for documenting care known as an ADL sheet.

- Use standard abbreviations.

- Incident reports are made and submitted separately and are not part of the chart.

*Hints in proper documentation:*

- Are all entries legible?

- Are there grammatical or spelling errors?

- Are entries signed correctly?

- Are entries dated and signed?

- Is the note free of erasures and other alterations?

- Are entries written in black ink?

## LEGAL ACCOUNTABILITY

- A nursing assistant is accountable for his or her actions, or in certain circumstances, omissions, when caring for a client or resident. He or she is accountable to the client, the medical team, peers, employer, and society at large.

- Once a nurse assistant assumes responsibility for the client or resident to exercise his or her professional skills, the nurse assistant owes the client a legal duty of care. He or she holds himself or herself out as possessing the qualifications, skills, and competence expected of the job.

- Inexperience is no defense to a claim of professional negligence. A CNA is expected to practice his or her skills according to the standard.

- The nursing assistant must keep up to date in his or her field of practice.

## CODE OF ETHICS FOR NURSING ASSISTANTS

### Technically Prepared

The learning and training process for CNAs does not end with the completion of the certification. There is a need to continuously update and advance one's competencies and technical skills in client care through in-service training and possibly continuing education.

### Personal Appearance

Nursing assistants' personal appearance is the manner they are observed by their co-workers, employers, and patients each day. Grooming and hygiene should be maintained regardless of personal situations. Conduct and facial gestures should be comforting and friendly to the clients and other colleagues.

### Patient Care

It's the duty of a CNA to work toward easing the pain and improving the health of the patient. Provide equal care to all patients, irrespective of their religion, race, gender, age, or medical condition. Along with medical needs, a nursing professional is also responsible to address the emotional, physical, spiritual, and social requirements of the patients.

### Personal Accountability

As a nursing aide, you should acknowledge responsibility for your behavior and actions. You should not work under the influence of drugs or alcohol; you must not be involved in falsification or alteration of records; and you should not exhibit unprofessional behavior. You are accountable for the following actions:

- Arriving on time.

- Displaying honesty and trustworthiness.

- Working well with a team and respecting colleagues.

- Following work-related guidelines.

- Honoring patient confidentiality.

**Health Insurance Portability and Accountability Act (HIPAA).**

According to HIPAA, health care professionals are not allowed to disclose or discuss a client's personal or health care information with anyone, except the caregivers and supervisors engaged in the patient's care. If the client's data is maintained on a computer, all the passwords, usernames and access codes should be kept secured and protected. In case of a breach of security, immediately inform your supervisor.

**High Level of Performance**

Nurse assistants should always try to render care services to the best of their ability. A patient's safety and welfare must be the first concern. Inform your immediate supervisor in case the patient care doesn't meet the desired standard of excellence.

- Observe the Code of Ethics.

- Be loyal to your co-workers, patients, and employer.

- Keep yourself in good health and practice healthy habits. Get sufficient sleep, eat a nutritious diet, and get periodic health check-ups.

- Never discuss your personal affairs and problems with the client.

- Never give or perform a treatment or procedure for which you are not qualified to perform.

- Be flexible and keen to accept changes in assignments and tasks necessary to improve the condition of the patient.

# MEMBER OF THE HEALTH CARE TEAM

## TERMS TO REMEMBER:

- **Chain of Command**: The authoritative structure established to resolve administrative, clinical, or other patient safety issues by allowing health care clinicians to present an issue of concern through the lines of authority until a resolution is reached.

- **Collaboration**: Working with another person or members in a health care group in order to achieve common goals and objectives of care.

- **Continuity of Care**: The process by which the patient and the members of the health care team are cooperatively involved in ongoing health care management toward the goal of high quality, cost-effective medical care.

- **Delegation**: Entrusting the performance of a selected nursing task to an individual who is qualified, competent, and able to perform such tasks. The one who delegates retains the accountability for the total nursing care of the individual.

- **Discharge Planning**: The activities that facilitate a patient's movement from one health care setting to another, or to home. It is a multidisciplinary process involving physicians, nurses, nursing assistants, LPNs, social workers, and other related health care professionals.

- **Line of Authority**: The line of authority, or also known as the chain of command is the structure of authority and responsibility through the medical team. Through the chain of command, certain members have the authority to task subordinate members to perform a task within their job description. However, just by ordering someone to perform the task, that person does not relinquish responsibility. The line of authority within a team or group establishes who is in charge of giving orders.

- **Policy**: A course of action that should be taken every time a certain situation occurs.

- **Procedure**: A particular method or way of doing something.

- **Teamwork**: A dynamic process involving two or more health care professionals with complementary backgrounds and skills, sharing common health goals and exercising concerted physical and mental effort in assessing, planning, or evaluating patient care.

## SKILLS TO BE MASTERED

- Collaborative skills

- Effective communication skills

- Performing delegated health care tasks

- Teaching reinforcement on client's or resident's care

- Referral skills to necessary personnel and settings

- Coordinating with client's support system

- Decision-making skills

- Proactive conflict resolution skills

- Teamwork

Nursing assistants are part of the health care professional team that includes physicians, nurses, social workers, therapists, dieticians, and specialists. In rendering health care service, all members of the team should focus on the client or resident. The team revolves around the client or resident and his or her condition, treatment, and progress. Each member has his or her own functions but the client or the resident remains the most important member of the team.

## CHAIN OF COMMAND

As a nursing assistant, you are carrying out instructions given to you by a nurse. The nurse is acting on the instructions of a physician or another member of the team. The chain of command helps guarantee that the client or resident is receiving the necessary services and also protects you, the team, and the employer from liability.

Understand what you can and cannot perform. These are indicated in the standard of CNA practice, facility policies, and contract. You are working under the license of another health care professional, e.g. charge nurse, who delegates the performance of certain tasks based on the scope of CNA practice.

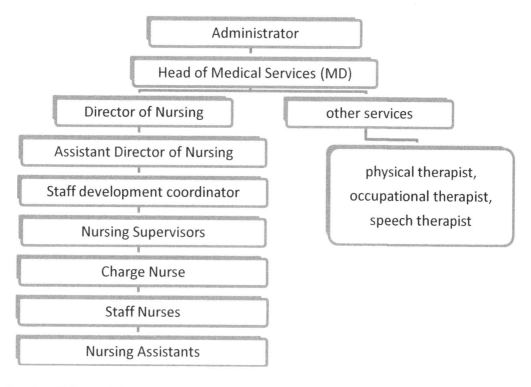

## Institutional Policies and Procedures

During the job orientation, the CNA will be given or will be made aware of the policies and procedures that all staff members are expected to follow. One example of a policy is adherence to the plan of care. A procedure can include a particular method for reporting information about clients or residents, e.g. what form to fill out, when and how often to fill it out, and to whom it is given.

*Common policies in nursing homes or long-term facilities:*

- Information given in client's contract with the facility or health care relationship must remain confidential.

- The client's or resident's plan of care must be followed accordingly.

- Avoid performing tasks that are not stipulated in the job description and scope of practice.

- Nursing assistants must report important events or changes in the client's or resident's condition to a nurse.

- Personal problems must not be discussed with the resident or the resident's family.

- Nursing assistants must be on time for work.

- As members of the team, nursing assistants must be dependable.

*Professional Practice Boundaries*

- Maintaining authenticity in all relationships with others such as CNA–to–CNA relationships, CNA-to-nurse relationships, CNA-to-patient relationships, and multidisciplinary collaboration.

- Addressing and evaluating issues of impaired practice, e.g. developing unprofessional relationships with clients or residents, accepting inappropriate gifts from clients and families, confidentiality and privacy violations, conducting illegal practices, and maintaining an unsafe environment.

*Self-care Boundaries and Obligations*

- Participating in self-care activities to maintain and promote moral self-respect, professional growth, and competence.

- Advancing knowledge through practice, education, and health care contributions as a member of the team.

- Collaborating with other health care team members and other health professionals to promote management efforts for the improvement and maintenance of quality services.

## DELEGATION

As a result of managed care and budget constraints, the delegation of health care tasks to CNAs has increased at a startling rate. Nurse assistants are performing increasingly complex tasks, and RNs, in turn, are undertaking increased responsibility for supervising the care CNAs provide.

When registered nurses delegate specific nursing functions or tasks to nursing assistants, they retain the responsibility and accountability to the public for the overall nursing care. CNAs are continuously being supervised and evaluated to determine their competencies in performing the needed tasks.

There are commonly accepted rules of delegation, which mandate that the delegated activity involves the:

- right task,

- right circumstances,

- right person,

- right communication, and

- right feedback

*What Can Be Delegated?*

It is important for the nursing assistants to understand appropriate activities and tasks that are acceptable to be delegated to them. It is the responsibility of the CNA to accept or refuse tasks according to his or her job description, scope of practice, and level of competencies or capabilities.

These delegated tasks typically are ones that:

- frequently occur,

- are considered technical by nature,

- are considered standard and unchanging,

- have predictable results, and

- have minimal potential for risks

*Alert:* If CNAs perform functions beyond their level of required competencies and practice, they can be criminally prosecuted for practicing nursing or medical interventions without a license. They should not practice beyond the parameters of recognized delegated functions.

## COLLABORATIVE HEALTH CARE

To deliver optimal health care to the client or resident, nurse assistants must work as productive members of the team providing comprehensive health care. Collaboration means a collegial relationship with other health care providers in the provision of client or patient care.

Collaborative practices include the discussion of patient diagnosis and cooperation in the management and delivery of care. Each collaborator is available to the other for consultation either in person or by communication device, but need not be always physically present on the premises at the time the actions are performed.

**The CNA as a Collaborator:**

Nursing assistants collaborate with CNA colleagues and other health care professionals. Education and training are integral to ensuring that the members of each professional group understand the collaborative nature of their roles, specific contributions, and the importance of working together. Each member needs to understand how an integral delivery system centers on the client's health care needs rather than on the particular care given by one group.

*CNA with Nurse Assistant Colleagues:*

- Shares personal expertise with other CNAs and elicits the expertise of others to ensure quality client care.

- Develops a sense of trust and mutual respect with other CNAs that recognizes their unique contributions.

*CNA with Other Health Care Professional Members:*

- Recognizes the contribution that each member of the interdisciplinary team can make by virtue of his or her expertise and view of the situation.

- Listens to each individual's views.

- Shares health care responsibilities in exploring options, setting goals, and making decisions with clients and families.

- Participates in collaborative interdisciplinary research to increase knowledge of a clinical problem or situation.

*CNA with Professional Health Organizations:*

- Seeks opportunities to collaborate with and within professional organizations.

- Serves on committees or specialty groups.

- Supports health care groups in actions to create solutions for professional and health care concerns.

**Competencies Basic to Collaboration**

- **Communication:** Collaborating to solve complex problems requires effective communication skills.

  - Effective communication can occur only if the involved parties are committed to understanding each other's professional roles and appreciating each other as individuals.

  - Sensitivity must be observed in dealing with differences in communication styles.

  - Members should center on their common ground of care: the client's or resident's needs.

- **Mutual Respect and Trust:** Mutual respect occurs when two or more people show or feel honor toward one another.

- Trust occurs when a person is confident in the actions of another person.

- Both mutual trust and respect imply a mutual process and must be expressed both verbally and nonverbally.

- **Decision Making:** All team members share responsibility for the outcome.

  - To create a solution, the team follows each step of the decision-making process starting with a clear definition of the problem.

  - It must be directed at the objectives of the specific effort.

  - Members must be able to verbalize their perspectives in a nonthreatening environment.

  - Focus on the client's or resident's priority needs and organizing interventions accordingly.

  - The discipline best able to address the client's needs is given priority in planning and is responsible for providing its interventions in a timely manner.

## TEAMWORK

Performing teamwork generally works better when members of the team have prior experience working together due to enhanced coordination and communication. The teamwork process involves the following steps:

- Transition processes (between periods of action)

  - Mission analysis

  - Goal specification

  - Strategy formulation

- Action processes (when the team attempts to accomplish its goals and objectives)

  - Monitoring progress toward goals

  - Systems monitoring

  - Team monitoring and backup behavior

  - Coordination

- Interpersonal processes (present in both action periods and transition periods)

- Conflict management

- Motivation and confidence building

- Affect management

*Benefits of Teamwork:*

- **Problem solving**: A single brain can't bounce different ideas off of itself. Each team member has a responsibility to contribute equally and offer their unique perspective on a problem to arrive at the best possible solution for the client or patient.

  - Teamwork can lead to better decisions or services.

  - The quality of teamwork may be measured by analyzing the following six components of collaboration among team members:

    1. Communication

    2. Coordination

    3. Balance of member contributions

    4. Mutual support

    5. Effort

    6. Cohesion

- **Developing relationships**: A health care team that continues to work together will eventually develop an increased level of bonding.

  - This can help people avoid unnecessary conflicts since they have become well acquainted with each other through teamwork.

  - Team members' ratings of satisfaction with their team are correlated with the level of teamwork processes present.

- **Everyone has unique qualities**: Every team member can offer their unique knowledge and ability to help improve other team members. Through teamwork, the sharing of these qualities will allow team members to be more productive in the future.

- **In healthcare**: Teamwork is associated with increased patient safety and promotes quality assurance in care.

## CONTINUITY OF CARE

Continuity of care is the coordination of health care services by health care providers for clients moving from one health care setting to another and between and among health care professionals.

*Alert:* Continuity ensures uninterrupted and consistent services for the client from one level of care to another. It maintains client-focused individualized care and helps optimize the client's health status.

To provide continuity of care, the nurse assistant needs to consider the following:

- Help in the implementation of the discharge planning initiated by the nurse for all clients when they are admitted in the facility.

- Involve the client and the client's family or support persons in the planning process.

- Collaborate with other health care professionals as needed to ensure that medical, psychosocial, cultural, and spiritual needs are met.

## REFERRALS

The referral process is a systematic problem-solving approach that helps clients to use resources that meet their health care needs. It involves knowledge of the community resources and an ability to solve problems, set priorities, coordinate, and collaborate.

Home care referrals are often made for the following clients:

- Elders

- Children with complex conditions

- Frail persons who live alone

- Those who lack or have a limited support system

- Those who have a caregiver whose health is failing

- Those whose home presents risks to their safety

# CLINICAL SKILLS TEST

## WHAT TO EXPECT?

The Clinical Skills Test (CST) is the second portion of the CNA certification examination. It is a clinical-based test where a CNA candidate demonstrates his or her knowledge and skills on practical training to prove that he or she has the necessary competencies required in performing the duties and responsibilities of a nursing assistant in the health care setting.

As a CNA candidate, you need to pass both the written and the clinical skills exams to complete the certification. Each clinical skill assessment is based on what you were trained on during your clinical skills training course. The skills part is by far the most important part of the exam, the most difficult, and carries the most weight. It is where the majority of those who fail to pass get their lowest performance in the entire test.

There are variations in the conduct of the CST from state to state depending on the area where you are taking the certification test.

- There might be some duties in one state that do not fall under the duties of a nursing assistant in another.

- In some areas, you might be asked to demonstrate only three different CNA skills, while most states will require five or six.

- Some CNA skills test will allow you to select the procedures to be demonstrated to the proctor, but most areas will require you to demonstrate certain skills at random.

An assigned examiner, a Registered Nurse, will select an average of five clinical skills for you to demonstrate within 35 to 45 minutes from a total of 25 to 30 skills. You will be graded accordingly in the different domains of your learning, which covers the cognitive, psychomotor, and affective areas or KSA (knowledge, skills, and attitude). The examiner is judging your overall knowledge (cognitive), competency in performing the procedures (psychomotor) and demeanor or attitude (affective) in the performance of the selected duties.

You will be required to perform the selected procedures on a dummy or an actual person who shall serve the patient. This is a simulation of the performance of your tasks in providing direct actual care to your clients in the practice of your profession. The selection of the clinical skills to be demonstrated can range from simple to the more complex ones, or usually a combination of the two.

The list of the 25 clinical skills commonly used by examiners was already provided to you in the early part of this study guide, but here they are again for reference:

1. Hand washing

2. Apply one knee-high elastic stocking or anti-embolic stocking

3. Assist to ambulate a client using transfer belt

4. Assist client with use of bedpan

5. Clean upper and lower dentures

6. Count and record client's radial pulse

7. Count and record patient's respirations

8. Don and remove gown and gloves (PPE)

9. Dress client with affected (weak) right arm

10. Feed client who cannot feed self

11. Give modified bed bath

12. Make an occupied bed

13. Measure and record blood pressure

14. Measure and record urinary output

15. Measure and record weight of ambulatory client

16. Perform passive range of motion exercises for client knee and ankle

17. Perform passive range of motion exercises for client shoulder

18. Position client on side

19. Provide catheter care for female client

20. Provide fingernail care

21. Provide food care

22. Provide mouth care

23. Provide perineal care for female client

24. Transfer from bed to wheelchair using transfer belt

25. Moving patient from bed to the stretcher

The details of most of the procedures can be found under the chapter of the Basic Nursing Skills. Additional skills that you may encounter can include the following:

- Assisting Residents Who Have Memory Loss, Confusion, or Understanding Problems

- Communicating With Residents Who Have Problems with Speech

- Communicating With the Hearing Impaired

- How to Start Conversations and Send Messages

## TIPS ON THE CST:

*Have the right attitude.*

- Demonstrate confidence and precision in the performance of the procedures.

  - Avoid unnecessary nervous mannerisms.

  - Talk clearly in a proper pace and tone. Nervousness can cause examinees to rush with their speech, mumble, or even stammer.

- Act like a real CNA in practice, not a newbie student in a training course.

- Show enthusiasm and warmth. Keep those smiles on.

*Learn proper stress management. Manage your anxiety level.*

- Prepare yourself physically. Have an adequate rest and a healthy meal before the test.

- Attend to your bladder needs before the test.

- Do relaxation techniques like proper breathing, guided imagery, or whatever works for you.

### Know what you are getting into. Do not go into the battle unarmed.

- Have a grasp of how the CST is being conducted.

- When you are preparing to take the CNA skills test, study all the materials you covered during your training course.

- Know the coverage of the test.

- Watch CNA training Classes demonstration videos and practice along before it is time to take your test.

- Consider other CNA examinees' experiences in the past. They can share brief concepts and you can also learn what worked or what didn't work for them.

### Develop a sense of focus.

- Not everything that you learned in the CNA course and trainings will come out in the exam. Know the commonly asked concepts and skills being tested.

- Create your own review timeline in mastering the different clinical skills.

- Have a checklist of the procedures you need to demonstrate.

### Master the common basic techniques throughout the test.

The test administrators want to see the nursing assistants demonstrate a common basic technique throughout the test. With all the clinical skills, you can easily get overwhelmed in your preparation. DO NOT UNDERESTIMATE THE BASICS. There are those who fail the exam because they've focused too much on the complex skills while forgetting the most basic ones. Master these first until they become second nature.

- Demonstrate sound direct care hygiene techniques such hand washing before making any contact as a standard precaution demonstrating sound infection control measures. Regardless of the skill you will be demonstrating, always remember to wash your hands.

- Keep in mind that the different skills usually have common procedural ways of starting and ending. Do not hesitate to repeat these in the succeeding skills that you will be asked to perform.

**Prior to demonstration of a skill:**

- Be sure you understand the task and ask questions or clarifications before starting.

- Check and prepare all the equipment you need. Ask the test administrator for any missing article. You will be demonstrating in an ideal setting where all the necessary materials are provided.

**If you are now asked to perform a skill, start with the following common guidelines:**

- Establish rapport. Inform the patient or the dummy of your presence. Greet him or her accordingly and address the patient by his or her name.

- Explain the procedure that you will be performing. Ask the patient if he or she has any questions or concerns regarding the procedure and be sure to elicit consent or permission before proceeding.

- Wash your hands thoroughly.

- Setup all the appropriate equipment ready for use.

- Prepare the patient for the procedure.

**At the end of every procedure, it is necessary to perform the following concluding steps:**

- Inform the patient that you are finished and ask him or her for concerns.

- Check that the patient or dummy is in a comfortable position and ensure safety.

- Properly stow the equipment and maintain overall sanitation of the room.

- Perform hand washing.

*Have a brush on communication skills.*

- Effective communication with the patient throughout the procedure will increase the subject's compliance and cooperation. Meeting the client's wishes or concerns demonstrates sound communication techniques.

- Even if you are performing on a dummy, talk to it like it is an actual patient needing the care you are rendering.

- The examiner will be evaluating indirect care that consists of interaction with the client, demonstrating communication skills.

### Always consider patient's safety.

- The examiner will ask you to demonstrate a position change of a client lying in bed from their back to their side. The examiner is looking at consideration of the client's safety such as not being placed or rolled close to the edge of the bed.

- You might also be asked to show the proper way to reposition a patient in order to prevent bedsores.

- Observe the use of proper body mechanics.

- Check the side rails of the bed.

### Do not forget the patient's privacy in demonstrating care.

- Always knock on the door before entering the room.

- Show the proper use of curtains and drapes in performing the necessary procedure.

- For bodily care such as personal hygiene, only expose body parts one at a time depending on the steps of the procedure, e.g. bed bath and perineal care.

### Maintain the patient's worth and dignity.

- This is reflected in the demonstration of skills with positive regard, allowing the patient to communicate needs, addressing the patient's concerns, providing privacy, and ensuring safety.

### Observe asepsis or basic infection control.

- Proper hand washing.

- Donning of personal protective equipment (PPE) such as gloves as needed depending on the procedure and case given.

- Proper removal of the PPE.

- Disposal of waste and maintaining environmental sanitation.

- Always be mindful of preventing the spread of infection or contamination from hand washing to the use of equipment and managing the patient's environment.

*Practice!*

Skills are not developed overnight. Don't expect to simply memorize the steps and then be able to perform them correctly all at once.

- Know your strengths and weaknesses in the performance of the different skills.

- Watch CNA training videos on the proper demonstration of the skills.

- **Do Role Playing.**

  - Ask someone, a friend or family member, to play the patient role while you practice with the performance of the skills.

  - Have another person serve as the test administrator as you perform under the pressure of a time constraint, grading system, and the consciousness of being watched and evaluated.

# CST FLASH CARDS

The following are Critical Skills Test Flash Cards to help you practice the necessary steps for your practical skills portion of the CNA Exam.

**When entering patient's room:**

1. Knock & wait

2. Introduce yourself

3. Pull privacy curtain

4. Explain procedure

**Common steps in beginning with a clinical skill:**

1. Prepare supplies.

2. Knock and wait

3. Introduce yourself to the patient,

4. Pull the Curtain,

5. Explain procedure

**Last three common steps of every clinical skill:**

1. Call light in hand

2. Bed locked & in lowest position

3. Wash hands

## Procedure: Hand Washing/ Hand Hygiene

1. Turn on sink water.

2. Wet hands with warm water and apply soap.

3. Lather all portions of the hand to include the wrists, fingers, cuticles, and under the nails. Use cuticle brush for the nails.

4. Perform above step for at least **20 seconds**.

5. Rinse hands with fingers lower than the wrists.

6. Dry your hands with paper towel.

7. Use a paper towel to turn off the water.

DO NOT TOUCH THE SINK AT ANYTIME.

## Procedure: Measuring Oral Body Temperature

1. Prepare thermometer.

2. Place a disposable plastic cover over the probe.

3. Ask patient of any recent intake of hot or cold beverage or food.

4. Open the patient's mouth.

5. Gently slide the probe to the back of the mouth under the tongue.

6. Ask the patient to close mouth and keep the probe in place.

7. Remove the thermometer from the patient's mouth.

8. Eject the disposable plastic cover into an appropriate waste basket.

9. Return the thermometer.

## Procedure: Measuring Rectal Body Temperature

1. Place patient in Sim's position and raise side rail.

2. Bare only the perineal area.

3. Remove the thermometer and attach a rectal probe to it.

4. Apply lubricant to the probe covering 1 to 2 inches.

5. Separate the patient's butt cheeks to expose the anus.

6. Inform patient of the probe ask him or her to breathe.

7. Gently insert the probe into the anus 1 to 2 inches deep.

8. Hold the thermometer in place while it takes its readings.

9. Slowly remove the probe from the anus.

10. Eject the disposable plastic cover into the appropriate trash.

11. Return the thermometer back.

12. Wipe the patient's anal area to remove lubricant and any other material.

13. Replace the patient's garments.

14. Assist patient back to a comfortable position.

**Procedure: Measuring Axillary Body Temperature**

1. Prepare thermometer.

2. Place a disposable plastic cover over the probe.

3. Position the patient sitting up or in a position of comfort.

4. Insert the thermometer probe into the center axilla.

5. Place the patient's arm down and across the chest.

6. Wait and take the reading.

7. Eject the disposable plastic cover into an appropriate wastebasket.

8. Return the thermometer back.

**Procedure: Measuring the Radial Pulse**

1. Place patient in supine or sitting position.

   a. Supine position: rest the arm along the side or fold it across chest.

   b. Sitting position: support arm on a flat surface.

2. Slightly extend wrist.

3. Place index and middle fingers along the groove on thumb side.

4. Press down to feel the pulse.

5. Check pulse strength:

6. Count the pulse for30 seconds. Then multiply by 2.

   a. Note: for irregularities in pulse, count for 60 seconds.

7. Record the strength, rhythm and rate.

**Pulse grade or strength:**

- pounding-bounding (+4),

- strong-brisk (+3),

- normal (+2),

- thready (+1),

- non-existent/ absent (0).

**Procedure: Measuring Apical Pulse**

1. Prepare clean stethoscope.

2. Place patient in a sitting or supine position.

3. Locate the apical pulse on the left chest wall at about the 4.5 to 5th left intercostal space.

4. Position the stethoscope on site.

5. Count the beats for 30 seconds. Then multiply beats by 2.

6. Place client to comfortable position and clean equipment.

7. Record the strength, rhythm and rate.

**Procedure: Partial Bed Bath**

1. Prepare all equipment within arms reach.

    a. Note: check water temperature.

2. Drape the patient exposing only areas being washed at a time.

3. Place a towel under the patient or limb.

4. Use a wet washcloth without soap and clean the face. With the eyes, begin with the inner canthus and then the outer canthus. Dry the face.

5. Wash the neck, arms, hands and chest with washcloth. Dry.

6. Turn patient turn on the side. Wash the back.

7. Apply lotion to the back in a smooth circular motion.

8. Clean perineal area.

    a. Note: Allow client to wash perineal area if able to do so. If not, change gloves then perform as needed.

9. Keep patient dry.

10. Assist to comfortable position.

**Procedure: Providing Indwelling Catheter Care**

1. Position patient.

2. Female: placed on back with knees bent

3. Male: Fowler's position or supine.

4. Position a waterproof pad under the midsection to separate area from the bed.

5. Expose perineal area.

6. Access urethral meatus for insertion site.

7. Female: Use non-dominant hand to separate the labia

8. Male: separate the foreskin from the tip of the penis.

9. Hold the penis at the shaft for the remainder of the procedure.

10. Insert the catheter.

11. Check the perineal area for color, swelling, or problems.

12. Cleanse the perineal area

13. Cleanse the catheter tubing from the area of insertion to the connective tubing.

14. Reposition patient and cover their perineal area.

15. Document care.

## Procedure: Applying Condom Catheter

1. Place the patient in Fowler's position.

2. Expose the perineal area.

3. Clean the area, especially around the tip.

4. Remove the coverings from the condom catheter's adhesive surface.

5. Place the catheter at the end of the penis.

6. Roll the sides of the catheter down the shaft towards the body.

7. Apply tape down the length of the catheter is a spiral motion.

8. Secure the catheter.

9. Connect the catheter to the drainage bag.

10. Tape the tubing to the inner thigh.

11. Hang the drainage bag to the bed frame.

12. Document care

**Procedure: Measuring Respiratory Rate**

1. Place patient in sitting or supine position.

2. Watch the rise and fall of chest.

3. Distract patient while counting respiration.

4. Count for 30 seconds, multiply by 2.

    a. Note: If it is abnormal count for 60 seconds.

5. Record results including pattern of breathing.

**Procedure: Measuring Blood Pressure**

1. Place patient in supine or sitting position.

2. Check appropriate size of BP cuff.

3. Note: cuff should cover 40-45% of the upper arm.

4. Locate brachial artery.

5. Wrap the cuff around arm at least 2 inches from elbow.

6. Put arm at the level of the heart.

7. Position stethoscope over the brachial artery.

8. Pump cuff to approximately 30 mmHg above the systolic pressure.

9. Release pressure at a rate of about 2-3 mmHg per second.

10. mark the point on the gauge when you hear the first beat.

11. Deflate the cuff until you absence of sound.

12. Allow the cuff to completely deflate and remove from the patient.

13. Place the patient back in a comfortable position.

## Procedure: Providing Oral Care

1. Place patient in Fowler's position.

2. Minimize wetting clothing.

3. Apply toothpaste to wet tooth brush.

4. Ask patient to open mouth.

5. Using a circular motion, scrub their teeth, tongue and gums.

6. Allow the patient to rinse mouth out. Dry the patient.

7. Check for any sores or bleeding.

8. Dispose bib if used.

## Procedure: Placing patient in Lateral or Sim's position

1. Lock the wheels of the bed.

2. Place side rails up

3. Have patient move towards you.

4. Lateral: Place opposite arm under the head and closest arm across the chest.

   a. Sim's: Place opposite arm behind.

5. Take leg nearest you and cross it over the other leg.

6. Place one hand on the hip closest to you and place the other hand on the shoulder.

7. Inform patient of what you are doing and roll them away from you.

8. Add a pillow between their legs and between their arm and chest

## Procedure: Placing patient in Prone Position

1. Lock the wheels of the bed.

2. Place side rails up

3. Have patient move towards you.

4. Place patient on the stomach.

5. Turn head to the side.

6. Place arms in upward position.

## Procedure: Placing patient in Supine Position

1. Lock the wheels of the bed.

2. Place side rails up

3. Have patient move towards you.

4. Place patient on the back with head straight.

5. Place arms to the side and legs straight.

6. Place a pillow behind head.

## Procedure: Placing patient in Fowler's position

1. Lock the wheels of the bed.

2. Place side rails up

3. With the patient in a supine position, raise the head of the bed to a specific degree as indicated.

   a. Low Fowler's: 30 degrees

   b. Semi-fowler's: 45 to 60 degrees

   c. Fowler's: 90 degrees

4. Ensure that the patient is comfortable and won't slip.

## Procedure: Placing patient in Orthopneic Position

1. Lock the wheels of the bed.

2. Place side rails up

3. Place patient in sitting position.

4. Place a pillow on top bed side table in front of the patient.

5. Have the patient lean forward with arms position in front

**Procedure: Transferring Patient with Gait-Belt**

1. Secure the Gait belt around the patients waste.

2. Place yourself in front of the patient

3. Position the patient's feet in between yours.

4. Inform patient you will be placing your hands on the gait belt then proceed.

5. Assist patient in standing up while using the gait belt to pull him or her up.

6. Move one of your hands to the side of the gait belt

7. Place the other at the back of the belt.

8. Begin assisting in ambulating when ready.

9. Safely return client to a chair or bed.

**Supplies Needed in Occupied Bed:**

- Top Sheet

- Bottom Sheet

- Privacy Sheet

- Bed Sheet

**Procedure: Making an Occupied Bed**

1. Check record and verify patient's current status

2. Adjust the bed's height

3. Place the privacy sheet over the patient

4. Remove the bedspread first and then the blanket by rolling them down

5. Dispose of the sheets appropriately

6. Lower the rail on the side in which you intend to begin working

7. Have the patient scout over to the side near you

8. Then have the patient roll to the other side (where the bed rail is up).

9. Take the mattress linen and fold it over top of itself until you reach the patient's back.

10. Tuck the sheet under their shoulders, mid section and feet.

11. Place new clean sheets over the exposed portion of the mattress starting with the corners of the bed

12. Roll the sheets towards the patient and tuck them under the patient. Have the patient roll towards you

13. Raise the bed arm rail and move over the other side of the bed

14. Removed the soiled linen

15. Place dirty linen into the correct receptacle

16. Begin pulling the clean linen fully across the bed and secure the corners

17. Assist the patient into a comfortable position

18. Place the top sheets overtop of the privacy sheet and tuck under the foot of the bed. Do the same for the comforter

19. Take the top edge of the top sheets, and create a cusp

20. Raise the bed rail

21. Have the patient raise their head and remove the pillow

22. Replace the pillowcase

23. Place the pillow back under the patient's head

24. Dispose of the dirty linen

Note: Check with your patient and ask if he or she needs anything. Check for any red spots or sores.

**Procedure: Transferring Patient from Bed to Stretcher**

1. Position the bed at a comfortable height.

2. Place stretcher next to the bed and lock the wheels

3. Cover the patient with a privacy sheet

4. Remove the tops sheets by rolling them down the bed

5. Loosen the bottom sheet

6. Lower the bed rail on your side

7. Ask other two personnel go to the other side of the bed and roll the edges of the bottom sheet towards the patient

8. Inform the patient that you will be moving them over to the stretcher

9. Coordinate with the other two helpers, grab the sides of the sheet and move the resident over to the stretcher

10. Check patient's comfort and safety

**Procedure: Applying Anti-embolic stocking**

1. Supine position (lying down in bed)

2. Turn stocking inside out

3. Pull over toe, foot & heel

4. Then pull up leg (no twists or wrinkles)

5. Call Light, Bed Locked & Lowest

**Procedure: Assisting patient to Bedpan**

1. Lower head of bed

2. Raise opposite bed rail

3. Put on gloves

4. Roll client toward rail

5. Place bedpan under buttocks

6. Discard gloves & wash hands

7. Raise head of bed

8. Toilet paper, instruct on hand wipes, & call light w/in reach. Ask to signal when finished.

9. Lower head of bed

10. Put on gloves

11. Put up rail & roll client while holding bedpan

12. Remove bedpan, empty in toilet, rinse empty in toilet, & place in dirty area

13. Remove gloves & wash hands

**Procedure: Denture Care**

1. Put on gloves

2. Line sink with wash cloth

3. Run lukewarm water

4. Put tooth paste on tooth brush

5. Brush dentures

6. Rinse cup & fill with water

7. Place dentures in cup

8. Clean up

## Procedure: Dressing Patient with Affected Right Arm

1. Give client choice of clothing

2. Remove gown from unaffected arm (left arm) 1st, then affected side (right arm)

3. Dress affected side (right arm) 1st, then unaffected side (left arm)

4. Place soiled linens in hamper

5. Call Light, Bed Locked & Lowest

## Procedure: Feeding A Patient

1. Pick up name card & ask patient to state name

2. Set bed to 45-90 degree or upright position

3. Clean patient's hands with wipes

4. Inform patient what foods are available & what they would like to try first

5. Offer one bite of each food, tell them what it is

6. Offer beverage at least once during meal

7. Wipe month & hands with wipes

8. Remove tray, place food in trash & tray in dirty area

9. Call Light, Bed Locked & Lowest Position, Open Curtain

10. Wash Hands

## Procedure: Measuring Urinary Output

1. Pour the contents from bedpan into measuring container over toilet

2. Close toilet lid and place container flat

3. Empty into toilet

4. Rinse bedpan & measuring container & pour rinse into toilet

5. Trash gloves

6. Wash hands

7. Record in cc's (30 cc's = 1 oz)

**Procedure: Taking Patient's weight**

1. Allow patient with shoes on

2. Walk to scale & set scale to zero

3. Stand on side and assist if needed

4. Determine weight

5. Stand to side and assist if needed

6. Record weight

**Procedure: ROM for Knee and Ankle**

1. Instruct patient to report pain during procedure

2. Support leg at knee & ankle when performing ROM for knee

3. Bend knee and then return leg to normal position three times

4. Support foot & ankle close to the bed while performing ROM for ankle

5. Push and pull foot towards head then foot down, toes pointing down three times

6. Call light, bed locked & lowest position, open curtain, wash hands

**Procedure: ROM for the Shoulder**

1. Instruct patient to report pain during procedure

2. Support arm at elbow & wrist while performing ROM on shoulder

3. Raises patient's straightened arm away from the side position upward towards head to ear level & return arm down to side of body three times

4. Move straightened arm away from the side of body to shoulder level & return to side of body three times

5. Call light, bed locked & lowest position, open curtain, wash hands

**Supplies: Fingernail Care**

- Water basin

- Towel

- Washcloth

- Stick

- Nail file

**Procedure: Fingernail Care**

1. Check water temperature

2. Put on gloves

3. Put fingernails in water

4. Clean under fingernail with stick wiping stick after each nail

5. Dry fingernails and file as needed

6. Dispose of stick & file

7. Empty, rinse, & dry basin and put in dirty area

8. Dispose of dirty linens

9. Trash gloves & wash hands

**Procedure: Foot Care**

Supplies: 1 chuck pad, 1 towel, 1 washcloth, soap, lotion, water basin

1. Check water temperature

2. Put on gloves

3. Place foot in water & apply soap to wet washcloth

4. Lift and wash foot, including between the toes

5. Rinse foot in water, including between the toes

6. Dry foot, including between the toes

7. Apply lotion on top and bottom of foot (NOT between toes) & dry off excess

8. Empty, rinse & dry basin

9. Dispose of dirty linens

10. Ttrash gloves & wash hands

# PRACTICE EXAM 1

This examination is a practice test that involves various areas in the CNA practice. The set is randomly designed in such a way that it includes questions from basic or easy category to complex or difficult questions.

- Read each question carefully and choose the best answer.

- You are given one minute per question. Spend your time wisely!

- Be sure to read the answers and rationale.

1. Clients or residents disclose information pertaining to their condition and at times including personal issues during person-to-person interactions. To whom can the nurse aide share the information regarding a client's progress?

    A.   To other clients in the unit who show concern to this client

    B.   To the client's family and friends

    C.   To anyone who inquires about the client's condition

    D.   To the members of the health care team on the next shift

2. An 85-year-old client in a nursing home tells the nursing assistant, "Because the doctor was so insistent, I signed the papers for that research study. Also, I was afraid he would not continue taking care of me.: Which client right is being violated?

    A.   Right not to be harmed

    B.   Right to full disclosure

    C.   Right of privacy and confidentiality

    D.  Right of self-determination

3. Although the client refused the procedure, the nurse assistant insisted and inserted the urinary catheter. The administrator of the facility decides to settle the lawsuit because the nurse assistant is most likely to be found guilty of which of the following?

    A.  An unintentional tort

    B.  Assault

    C.  Invasion of privacy

    D.  Battery

4. The primary care provider wrote a do not resuscitate (DNR) order. The nurse assistant recognizes that which of the following applies in the care of the client?

    A.  The client may no longer make decisions regarding his or her own care

    B.  The client and the family know that the client will most likely die within the next 48 hours

    C.  The team will continue to implement all care focused on comfort and symptom management

    D.  A DNR order from a previous admission is valid for the current admission

5. The nurse assistant's spouse undergoes surgery at the hospital where the nurse assistant is employed. Which of the following practices is most appropriate?

    A.  Because the nurse assistant is an employee, access to the chart is allowed

    B.  The relationship with the client provides the nurse assistant special access to the chart

    C.  Access to the chart requires a signed release form

    D.  The nurse assistant can ask the surgeon to discuss the outcome of the surgery

6. The nurse assistant notices that a colleague's behaviors have changed during the past month. All of the following behaviors could indicate signs of impairment EXCEPT?

    A.  Increased absences from the unit during the shift

    B.  Interacts well with others

    C.  "Forgets" to sign out for obtaining articles

D. Administering drugs ordered to clients beyond her scope of practice

7. When an ethical issue arises, one of the most important responsibilities in managing client care situations is which of the following?

A. Be able to defend the morality of one's own actions

B. Remain neutral and detached when making ethical decisions

C. Ensure that the team is responsible for deciding ethical questions

D. Follow the client and family wishes exactly

8. CNAs are employed indifferent health care settings caring for clients with varied conditions. If a CNA is employed in a skilled nursing facility, he or she is serving in a:

A. Hospital

B. Rehabilitation center

C. Hospice center

D. Nursing home

9. Mrs. X, a 76-year-old client, is recovering from stroke. After being discharged from the hospital, clients, particularly of older people like her case, will be referred to what kind of health care facility?

A. Hospice facility

B. Subacute care center

C. Group or communal home

D. Respite facility

10. Assistive devices are necessary to help clients ambulate. When assisting a client in learning to use a walker, it is important to:

A. put padding all the way around the top rim.

B. let him walk by himself so he gains independence.

C. stand behind him and use a transfer belt.

D.  let him practice using the walker on the day he is discharged.

11. The nurse aide is monitoring the urine of a resident with minimal output. He may be suffering from urinary retention. Urinary retention refers to

A.  a normal output of urine.

B.  incontinence.

C.  a large output of urine.

D.  an inability to urinate.

12. In caring for elder clients, you need to be aware of the normal age-related changes. Normal hearing loss in aging known as presbycusis, is usually related to the difficulty in the ability to hear

A.  loud sounds.

B.  all sounds.

C.  high-pitched sounds.

D.  rapid speech.

13. Before providing any care, you have assure the identity of your client. Which one is considered the best way to safely identify your client?

A.  checking the name tag.

B.  ask him or her to state name.

C.  calling his name and waiting for his response.

D.  checking the bed plate.

14. After optimal recovery from spinal injury, Mr. Jack is placed on a bowel and bladder training program. He has not had a bowel movement for more than two days. What should the nurse aide do?

A.  Give the patient an enema.

B.  Offer prune juice.

C.  Increase fluids.

D.  Report it to the nurse in charge.

15. Following a motor vehicle accident, the parents refuse to permit withdrawal of life support from the child with no apparent brain function. The nurse assistant supports their decision. Which moral principle provides the basis for the nurse assistant's actions?

A.  Respect for autonomy

B.  Nonmaleficence

C.  Beneficence

D.  Justice

16. After recovering from hip replacement, an elderly client wants to go home. The family wants the client to go to a nursing home. If the nurse assistant is acting as a client advocate, the nurse assistant would:

A.  Inform the family that the client has the right to decide on her own.

B.  Ask the primary health care provider and nurse to discharge the client to home.

C.  Suggest the client to hire a lawyer to protect her rights

D.  Help the client and the family to communicate their views to each other.

17. Care in the home is an alternative to hospital placement. Which of the following is one major difference associated with in-home care?

A.  Does not focus on curative and life saving approaches

B.  Is less able to manage complex symptoms

C.  Facilitates extensive involvement of significant others or family

D.  Permits use of pain medication regimens not allowed in the hospital

18. If a primary care provider prescribed the following, which one can be delegated to a home nurse aide?

A.  Feeding and bathing the client

B.  Teaching the client about medications

C.  Assessing wound healing progress

D. Adjusting oxygen flow

19. A home health nurse assistant is providing care for a client who has paralysis on one side and whose spouse provides most of the care. which of the following may be a sign of caregiver role strain?

A. The caregiver losses weight and has insomnia

B. The caregiver asks other family and friends for help

C. The caregiver asks the nurse assistant and nurse what other ways he or she can help the client

D. The caregiver seems sad whenever the client's prognosis is discussed

20. The proper medical abbreviation for before meals is

A. PC

B. BID

C. OS.

D. AC

21. Upon taking the resident's blood pressure, the reading is 140/90 mmHg. The nurse aide considers the reading unusual. The proper medical term for high blood pressure is

A. Hypertension.

B. Tachycardia

C. Hypotension

D. Heart failure

22. A resident who has dysphagia or difficulty chewing or swallowing will be on what type of diet?

A. NPO

B. clear liquid diet

C. full liquid diet.

D. mechanically soft diet

23. Mrs Jackson, an 84-year-old resident diagnosed with dementia of the Alzheimer's type is found wandering around. She claims she cannot find her room. What should the nurse assistant do to promote Mrs. Jackson's independence?

    A.  Confront her and insist to her to stay in her room.

    B.  Ask a family member to watch her.

    C.  Place a familiar object outside her room door.

    D.  Write the room number on a piece of paper.

24. Aside from the vital signs, nurse aide also monitors the intake and output of the client on a regular basis. How often should a client's intake and output records be totaled?

    A.  every shift

    B.  twice a day

    C.  every four hours

    D.  every 12 hours

25. Which of the following should you observe and record when admitting a client?

    A.  bruises, marks, rashes, lesions or broken skin

    B.  color of the stool and amount of urine voided

    C.  when and how much the client has eaten and drunk

    D.  insurance policy information

26. The principles of prioritizing patient needs are grounded on several models of care. The Hierarchy of Human Needs is proposed by which of the following theorists?

    A.  Jean Piaget

    B.  Sigmund Freud

    C.  Abraham Maslow

    D.  Halbert Dunn

27. In reviewing Maslow's Hierarchy of needs, the client's needs are divided into different levels or hierarchy, namely:

    A. Assessment, diagnosis, planning, implementation and evaluation

    B. Physical, mental, social, spiritual

    C. Airway, breathing, circulation, nutrition, elimination

    D. Physiologic needs, safety and security, love and belongingness, self-esteem, and self-actualization

28. When responding to a client on the intercom, which of the following is the most appropriate response as a professional?

    A. ask the client, "Kindly state your name."

    B. say, "What do you want?"

    C. give your name and position and say, "May I help you?"

    D. say, "Please wait, the nurse will answer your call."

29. Mr. Greene is a newly admitted client in your unit. Which of the following things should you do to familiarize a new client with his environment?

    A. Tell Mr. Greene to refrain from operating the TV and other personal gadgets in the room.

    B. Show Mr. Greene where the call light is and how it works .

    C. Ask the visitors to leave the room until after admitting and orienting the client.

    D. Raise the side rails of the bed and raise the bed to high position.

30. Maintaining a safe environment is part of the functions of a CNA. When arranging a client's room, you should do all of the following EXCEPT

    A. administer medications as ordered on time.

    B. check signal cords.

    C. adjust the back and knee rests as directed.

    D. check lighting.

31. Its is important to practice standard precautions when

    A.  Providing oral hygiene

    B.  Dressing a client

    C.  Feeding a client

    D.  Ambulating a client

32. Mr. Harrington is scheduled for cleansing enema this morning. What position should a client be in to receive an enema ?

    A.  Semi-Fowler's

    B.  Lithotomy

    C.  Left Sim's

    D.  Prone

33. Rapid heart rate, rapid breathing, and dry mouth are examples of which of the following categories of signs and symptoms of stress:

    A.  Physical

    B.  Emotional

    C.  Cognitive

    D.  Affective

34. Those methods of disease treatment or prevention that are outside conventional practices are called:

    A.  Castigo de Dios

    B.  Yin and Yang

    C.  Shaman

    D.  Folk medicine

35. From the following, choose the phrase(s) that is/are true regarding the way in which an individual demonstrates pride in one's ethnicity

   A.   Placing value on specific physical characteristics

   B.   Giving one's children ethnic names

   C.   Wearing special items of clothing

   D.   All of the above are true statements

36. When developing a therapeutic relationship, a desired outcome is:

   A.   Developing a friendship

   B.   Making the client comfortable

   C.   Moving toward restoring health

   D.   Learning to know oneself

37. An example of verbal communication is:

   A.   Moaning

   B.   Laughing

   C.   Writing

   D.   Crying

38. An example of nonverbal communication is:

   A.   Speaking

   B.   Moaning

   C.   Reading

   D.   Writing

39. An obstacle to effective communication would be:

   A.   Using the principles of touch by giving the client a back rub

B.   Accepting what the client says while being alert to what he or she is not saying

C.   Asking the client if he or she feels lonely or sad

D.   Interrupting the client when he or she seems to be deep in thought

40. When the nurse assistant stops in during the evening, Mrs. D. states that she is very worried about her operation tomorrow. Of the following responses, which would be the most appropriate:

A.   "That is very understandable, Mrs. D., would you like to talk about your operation?"

B.   "Don' worry- everything is going to be okay."

C.   "That's just a routine operation that you are having. No need to worry about it."

D.   "You'll be okay- your doctor and our operating room staffs do these procedures every day."

41. It is suggested that the nurse sit in a relaxed position at eye level with the client when communicating with him or her because:

A.   This indicates that the nurse is fully involved in what is being communicated

B.   If the client feels rushed, he or she may interpret this to be disinterest by the nurse

C.   Responses to stress are manifested through active listening on the part of the nurse

D.   People have less control over nonverbal communication than they do over verbal communication

42. For the visual impaired client, it is easier to read:

A.   Large print in black ink on white paper

B.   Small print in black ink on white paper

C.   Large print in blue ink on off-white glossy paper

D.   Small print in blue ink on off-white glossy paper

43. For the hearing impaired client, the nurse can facilitate communication by:

A.   Talking louder, using simple words, and lowering voice pitch

B.   Sitting or standing beside the client's "bad" ear when talking

    C.  Selecting words that do not begin with the letters F, S, or K

    D.  Raising the voice pitch, talking softly, and repeating the words

44. Entries on the client's record should be objective, accurate, and legible because:

    A.  The client records are used by all health personnel in the health agency

    B.  The client's record are the property of the health agency and must be kept neat

    C.  The client has a right to read his or her chart; therefore, it must be legible and accurate

    D.  The client records are admissible as evidence in courts of law

45. Of the following individuals, which one is most likely to have a higher-than-average temperature?

    A.  The person experiencing apathy and depression

    B.  The person experiencing an average day

    C.  The person experiencing anxiety and nervousness

    D.  The person routinely working the night shift

46. The condition in which a person is aware of his or her own heart contraction without having to feel the pulse is called:

    A.  Arrhythmia

    B.  Pulse rhythm

    C.  Dysrhythmia

    D.  Palpitation

47. The total amount of water that most adults consume each day is:

    A.  1200-1500 mL/day

    B.  1500-2500 mL/day

    C.  1000-2000 mL/day

    D.  2000-3000 mL/day

48. The oral hygiene practice recommended to break up bacteria lodged between the teeth is:

    A.  Using dental floss between the teeth

    B.  Directing a jet spray between the teeth

    C.  Rinsing the mouth vigorously with a mouthwash

    D.  Using an electric toothbrush regularly

49. The term partial bath refers to:

    A.  Washing the area around the client's genitals and rectum only

    B.  Washing in a manner to remove secretions and excretions from less-soiled to more-soiled areas

    C.  Washing areas of the body that are subject to the greatest soiling or odor

    D.  Washing all areas of the body at the sink in the client's room

50. The first measure the nurse assistant must carry out when a fire occurs is:

    A.  Notifying the switchboard using the proper code

    B.  Turning off the oxygen supply near the fire

    C.  Using the appropriate fire extinguisher

    D.  Evacuating the people from the room with the fire

# PRACTICE EXAM 1 ANSWERS AND RATIONALE

1. Clients or residents disclose information pertaining to their condition and at times including personal issues during person-to-person interactions. To whom can the nurse aide share the information regarding a client's progress?

    A.   To other clients in the unit who show concern to this client

    B.   To the client's family and friends

    C.   To anyone who inquires about the client's condition

    D.   To the members of the health care team on the next shift

    ANSWER: D.

    RATIONALE: All information about a client from his or her diagnosis, treatment regimen to personal matters are part of privilege communication which can only be divulged to other members of the health care team who are directly related to his or her care.

    AREA: Client's rights

2. An 85-year-old client in a nursing home tells the nursing assistant, "Because the doctor was so insistent, I signed the papers for that research study. Also, I was afraid he would not continue taking care of me.: Which client right is being violated?

    A.   Right not to be harmed

    B.   Right to full disclosure

    C.   Right of privacy and confidentiality

    D.   Right of self-determination

    ANSWER:D. Right of self-determination

RATIONALE: The right of self-determination means that subjects feel free of constraints, coercion, or any undue influence to participate in a study

AREA: Client's/Patient's Rights

3. Although the client refused the procedure, the nurse assistant insisted and inserted the urinary catheter. The administrator of the facility decides to settle the lawsuit because the nurse assistant is most likely to be found guilty of which of the following?

A. An unintentional tort

B. Assault

C. Invasion of privacy

D. Battery

ANSWER: D. Battery

RATIONALE: Battery is the willful touching of a person without permission. Another name for unintentional tort is malpractice. This situation is intentional tort because the nurse assistant executed the act on purpose. Assault is the attempt or threat to touch another person unjustifiably or without permission. Invasion of privacy injures the feelings of a person and does not take into consideration how revealing information or exposing the client will affect the client's feelings.

AREA: Legal and Ethical Behavior

4. The primary care provider wrote a do not resuscitate (DNR) order. The nurse assistant recognizes that which of the following applies in the care of the client?

A. The client may no longer make decisions regarding his or her own care

B. The client and the family know that the client will most likely die within the next 48 hours

C. The team will continue to implement all care focused on comfort and symptom management

D. A DNR order from a previous admission is valid for the current admission

ANSWER: C. The team will continue to implement all care focused on comfort and symptom management

RATIONALE: A DNR order only controls CPR and similar lifesaving treatments. All other care continues as previously ordered. Competent clients can still decide about their own (including the DNR order). Nothing about the DNR order is related to when the client may die. Because clients' medical conditions and their viewsof their lives can change, a new DNR order is required for each admission to a health care agency. once admitted, that order stands until changed or until expires according to agency policy.

AREA: Legal and Ethical Behavior

5. The nurse assistant's spouse undergoes surgery at the hospital where the nurse assistant is employed. Which of the following practices is most appropriate?

A.   Because the nurse assistant is an employee, access to the chart is allowed

B.   The relationship with the client provides the nurse assistant special access to the chart

C.   Access to the chart requires a signed release form

D.   The nurse assistant can ask the surgeon to discuss the outcome of the surgery

ANSWER: C. Access to the chart requires a signed release form

RATIONALE: The only person entitled to information without written consent is the client and those providing direct care. the nurse assistant has open access to information regarding assigned clients only.

AREA: Legal and Ethical Behavior

6. The nurse assistant notices that a colleague's behaviors have changed during the past month. All of the following behaviors could indicate signs of impairment EXCEPT?

A.   Increased absences from the unit during the shift

B.   Interacts well with others

C.   "Forgets" to sign out for obtaining articles

D.   Administering drugs ordered to clients beyond her scope of practice

ANSWER: B. Interacts well with others

RATIONALE: Interacting with others (versus isolating self from others)and setting limits on the number of hours working are positive behaviors and not indicative of possible impairment. The other options are warning signs for impairment.

AREA: Legal and Ethical Behavior

7. When an ethical issue arises, one of the most important responsibilities in managing client care situations is which of the following?

A. Be able to defend the morality of one's own actions

B. Remain neutral and detached when making ethical decisions

C. Ensure that the team is responsible for deciding ethical questions

D. Follow the client and family wishes exactly

ANSWER: A. Be able to defend the morality of one's own actions

RATIONALE: A health care worker's actions in an ethical dilemma must be defensible according to moral and ethical standards. The nurse may have strong personal beliefs but distancing oneself from the situation does not serve the client. A team is not always required to reach decisions and the nurse assistant is not obliged to follow the client's wishes automatically when they may have negative consequences for self or others.

AREA: Legal and Ethical Behavior

8. CNAs are employed indifferent health care settings caring for clients with varied conditions. If a CNA is employed in a skilled nursing facility, he or she is serving in a:

A. Hospital

B. Rehabilitation center

C. Hospice center

D. Nursing home

ANSWER: D. Nursing Home

RATIONALE: A nursing home, convalescent home, skilled nursing facility (SNF), care home, rest home or intermediate care facility provides a type of residential care. It is a place of residence for people who require, as determined by a local hospital social worker and their nursing facility provider, continual nursing care and have significant difficulty coping with the required activities of daily living. Nursing aides and skilled nurses are usually available 24 hours a day, and most are large congregate care facilities with government funding. These facilities are supplemental or competing classes to home care, home health, community services-non-facility, and home and community-based Medicaid waiver services.

AREA: CNA as a member of the Health Care Team

9. Mrs. X, a 76-year-old client, is recovering from stroke. After being discharged from the hospital, clients, particularly of older people like her case, will be referred to what kind of health care facility?

A. Hospice facility

B. Subacute care center

C. Group or communal home

D. Respite facility

ANSWER: B. Subacute care center

RATIONALE: Subacute care center is a facility providing comprehensive inpatient care designed for someone who has an acute illness, injury, or exacerbation of a disease process. It is goal oriented treatment rendered immediately after, or instead of, acute hospitalization to treat one or more specific active complex medical conditions or to administer one or more technically complex treatments, in the context of a person's underlying long-term conditions and overall situation. It is generally more intensive than traditional nursing facility care and less intensive than acute care. in the case of Mrs. X, she will be needing additional continuous health care for the necessary follow up treatment or therapies to help her gain optimum function or to prevent further deterioration.

AREA: CNA as a member of the health care team

10. Assistive devices are necessary to help clients ambulate. When assisting a client in learning to use a walker, it is important to:

A. put padding all the way around the top rim.

B. let him walk by himself so he gains independence.

C. stand behind him and use a transfer belt.

D. let him practice using the walker on the day he is discharged.

ANSWER: C. stand behind him and use a transfer belt

RATIONALE: Standing behind him and using a transfer belt protects both the client and the aide. The client should be given adequate time to learn the use of the walker, to gain balance prior to discharge.

AREA: Restorative Skills

11. The nurse aide is monitoring the urine of a resident with minimal output. He may be suffering from urinary retention. Urinary retention refers to

A.  a normal output of urine.

B.  incontinence.

C.  a large output of urine.

D.  an inability to urinate.

ANSWER: D. an inability to urinate

RATIONALE: Urinary retention refers to an inability to urinate. Retention of urine is a symptom that should be reported to the charge nurse as soon as it is noted. In incontinence, the resident urinate more often with higher urine output with inability to control micturition.

AREA: Basic Nursing Skills

12. In caring for elder clients, you need to be aware of the normal age-related changes. Normal hearing loss in aging known as presbycusis, is usually related to the difficulty in the ability to hear

A.  loud sounds.

B.  all sounds.

C.  high-pitched sounds.

D.  rapid speech.

ANSWER: C. High-pitched sounds

RATIONALE: Because of this aspect of hearing loss, the aged hear well if you lower your voice. Shouting in a high-pitched voice does not help.

AREA: Restorative Skills

13. Before providing any care, you have assure the identity of your client. Which one is considered the best way to safely identify your client?

A. checking the name tag.

B. ask him or her to state name.

C. calling his name and waiting for his response.

D. checking the bed plate.

ANSWER: A. Checking the name tag

RATIONALE: The most accurate way of identifying a client is through his name band or tag. A confused patient may answer to any name or lie down in any bed. The next most accurate is asking him or her to state full name. Then if these means cannot be done, ask a third person to give the identity of the client with two additional personal identifiers or information about the client.

AREA: Basic Nursing Skills

14. After optimal recovery from spinal injury, Mr. Jack is placed on a bowel and bladder training program. He has not had a bowel movement for more than two days. What should the nurse aide do?

A. Give the patient an enema.

B. Offer prune juice.

C. Increase fluids.

D. Report it to the nurse in charge.

ANSWER: D. Report it to the nurse in charge

RATIONALE: The case should be reported to the charge nurse for the necessary additional assessment and management. Nurse Increasing fluids needs order in this case before implementation. The nurse aide is not allowed to give the client enema.

AREA: Restorative Skills

15. Following a motor vehicle accident, the parents refuse to permit withdrawal of life support from the child with no apparent brain function. The nurse assistant supports their decision. Which moral principle provides the basis for the nurse assistant's actions?

    A.  Respect for autonomy

    B.  Nonmaleficence

    C.  Beneficence

    D.  Justice

    ANSWER: A. Respect for autonomy

    RATIONALE: Autonomy is the client's (or surrogate's) right to make his or her own decision. The nurse assistant is obliged to respect the client's or significant other's informed decision. These parents may modify their decision as time goes on and the child's condition, or their feelings may change. This situation is not clearly one of nonmaleficence (do no harm) or beneficence (do good) since there are many aspects of both. If the child appeared to be suffering or an effective treatment is denied, these principles might apply. justice (fairness) generally applies when the rights of one client is being balanced against those of another client.

    AREA: Clients Rights

16. After recovering from hip replacement, an elderly client wants to go home. The family wants the client to go to a nursing home. If the nurse assistant is acting as a client advocate, the nurse assistant would:

    A.  Inform the family that the client has the right to decide on her own.

    B.  Ask the primary health care provider and nurse to discharge the client to home.

    C.  Suggest the client to hire a lawyer to protect her rights

    D.  Help the client and the family to communicate their views to each other.

    ANSWER: D. Help the client and the family to communicate their views to each other

    RATIONALE: A major role of the client advocate is to mediate between conflicting parties. The nurse assistant needs to check the situation further before offering any action. Informing the family is an intervention without assessment. If the primary health care provider sends the client home, the nurse assistant has not acted in resolving or reducing the conflict. Legal action should be a last resort.

AREA: Clients Rights

17. Care in the home is an alternative to hospital placement. Which of the following is one major difference associated with in-home care?

A. Does not focus on curative and life saving approaches

B. Is less able to manage complex symptoms

C. Facilitates extensive involvement of significant others or family

D. Permits use of pain medication regimens not allowed in the hospital

ANSWER: C. Facilitates extensive involvement of significant others or family

RATIONALE: Although hospitals have recently become more welcoming to families, a major strength of home care is the involvement and proximity of loved ones. Curative and lifesaving approaches may be used both at home and in the hospital. An asset of health care workers is their ability to manage more complex symptoms.

AREA: Member of the Health Care Team

18. If a primary care provider prescribed the following, which one can be delegated to a home nurse aide?

A. Feeding and bathing the client

B. Teaching the client about medications

C. Assessing wound healing progress

D. Adjusting oxygen flow

ANSWER: A. Feeding and bathing the client

RATIONALE: Assuming the client is medically stable, feeding and bathing are tasks within the aide's abilities. Teaching the client about medications, oxygen and performing assessments are duties restricted to the registered nurse.

AREA: Member of the Health Care Team

19. A home health nurse assistant is providing care for a client who has paralysis on one side and whose spouse provides most of the care. which of the following may be a sign of caregiver role strain?

   A.  The caregiver losses weight and has insomnia

   B.  The caregiver asks other family and friends for help

   C.  The caregiver asks the nurse assistant and nurse what other ways he or she can help the client

   D.  The caregiver seems sad whenever the client's prognosis is discussed

   ANSWER: A. The caregiver losses weight and has insomnia

   RATIONALE: If the caregiver's own health is becoming threatened, it may be a sign of overload. It would be appropriate for the caregiver to ask for assistance or ask for clarification of ways he or she can assist the client. Sadness related to a poor prognosis would be a normal and expected response as long as it does not evolve to depression.

   AREA: Emotional and Mental Health Needs

20. The proper medical abbreviation for before meals is

   A.  PC

   B.  BID

   C.  OS.

   D.  AC

   ANSWER: D. AC

   RATIONALE: The proper medical abbreviation for before meals is AC or antecebum. PC, post cebum is after meals, BID means twice a day and OS, Occulosinistre, refers to left eye.

   ANSWER: Communication

21. Upon taking the resident's blood pressure, the reading is 140/90 mmHg. The nurse aide considers the reading unusual. The proper medical term for high blood pressure is

   A.  Hypertension.

   B.  Tachycardia

C. Hypotension

D. Heart failure

ANSWER: A. Hypertension

RATIONALE: High blood pressure is referred to as hypertension. Abnormally low blood pressure is hypotension. Tachycardia is abnormally rapid or high pulse rate. Heart failure is pump failure where the heart fails to adequate blood for circulation.

AREA: Basic Nursing Skills

22. A resident who has dysphagia or difficulty chewing or swallowing will be on what type of diet?

A. NPO

B. clear liquid diet

C. full liquid diet.

D. mechanically soft diet

ANSWER: D. Mechanically soft diet

RATIONALE: A mechanical soft diet is easy to chew, swallow, and digest. It is easier to swallow soft diet than liquid. NPO or nothing per orem, nothing by mouth is usually indicated before and immediately after major surgical operation.

AREA: Basic Nursing skill

23. Mrs Jackson, an 84-year-old resident diagnosed with dementia of the Alzheimer's type is found wandering around. She claims she cannot find her room. What should the nurse assistant do to promote Mrs. Jackson's independence?

A. Confront her and insist to her to stay in her room.

B. Ask a family member to watch her.

C. Place a familiar object outside her room door.

D. Write the room number on a piece of paper.

ANSWER: C. Place a familiar object outside her room door

RATIONALE: Dementia is characterized by progressive decline in cognitive function such as memory and motor abilities. The client needs to be reoriented regularly to her surroundings. Use the 4 Cs to alleviate confusion: clock, calendar, color, codes. Helping her locate her room on her own with the guide can help her have a sense of control and makes her feel good about herself.

AREA: Restorative Skill

24. Aside from the vital signs, nurse aide also monitors the intake and output of the client on a regular basis. How often should a client's intake and output records be totaled?

A.  every shift

B.  twice a day

C.  every four hours

D.  every 12 hours

ANSWER: A. every shift

RATIONALE: Input and output are totaled once per shift as well as every 24 hours.

AREA: Basic Nursing Skills

25. Which of the following should you observe and record when admitting a client?

A.  bruises, marks, rashes, lesions or broken skin

B.  color of the stool and amount of urine voided

C.  when and how much the client has eaten and drunk

D.  insurance policy information

ANSWER: A. bruises, marks, rashes, lesions or broken skin

RATIONALE: On gross observation and inspection, the nurse aide can readily check the client's skin integrity, mood, gross appearance and hygiene. Although all of these can be included in the admission assessment, the presence of injuries is of the highest priority which may necessitate further investigation, reporting and immediate management. Failure to notice bruises or marks on the skin on admission may later cause someone to believe you were involved in abuse.

AREA: Basic Nursing Skill

26. The principles of prioritizing patient needs are grounded on several models of care. The Hierarchy of Human Needs is proposed by which of the following theorists?

A. Jean Piaget

B. Sigmund Freud

C. Abraham Maslow

D. Halbert Dunn

ANSWER: C. Abraham Maslow

RATIONALE: Maslow's hierarchy of needs is a theory in psychology proposed by Abraham Maslow in his 1943 paper "A Theory of Human Motivation". Halbert Dunn'stheory focuses on the attainment of high level of wellness. Sigmund Freud developed the Psychosexual and Psychoanalytic theory while Jean Piaget described the different stages of cognitive development.

AREA: Basic Nursing Skills

27. In reviewing Maslow's Hierarchy of needs, the client's needs are divided into different levels or hierarchy, namely:

A. Assessment, diagnosis, planning, implementation and evaluation

B. Physical, mental, social, spiritual

C. Airway, breathing, circulation, nutrition, elimination

D. Physiologic needs, safety and security, love and belongingness, self-esteem, and self-actualization

ANSWER: D. Physiologic needs, safety and security, love and belongingness, self-esteem, and self-actualization

RATIONALE: Maslow's hierarchy of needs is often portrayed in the shape of a pyramid with the largest, most fundamental levels of needs at the bottom and the need for self-actualization at the top. The layers of needs according to priority are: Physiological needs, safety, love and belonging, esteem and self-actualization. The most basic needs must be met first before the client achieves the succeeding higher needs in the hierarchy.

AREA: Basic Nursing Skills

28. When responding to a client on the intercom, which of the following is the most appropriate response as a professional?

    A.  ask the client, "Kindly state your name."

    B.  say, "What do you want?"

    C.  give your name and position and say, "May I help you?"

    D.  say, "Please wait, the nurse will answer your call."

    ANSWER: C. give your name and position and say, "May I help you?"

    RATIONALE: When responding to a patient on the intercom, you should give your name and position. This allows for orientation for the client of the health care team member on the line as well as the role or position with the interest to address his or her concerns.

    AREA: Communication

29. Mr. Greene is a newly admitted client in your unit. Which of the following things should you do to familiarize a new client with his environment?

    A.  Tell Mr. Greene to refrain from operating the TV and other personal gadgets in the room.

    B.  Show Mr. Greene where the call light is and how it works .

    C.  Ask the visitors to leave the room until after admitting and orienting the client.

    D.  Raise the side rails of the bed and raise the bed to high position.

    ANSWER: B. Show Mr. Greene where the call light is and how it works

    RATIONALE: You should never leave a newly admitted client until he or she knows how to call for help. Orient the client to the unit and the team. The client can watch the television and can use personal gadgets as long as these equipments to not interfere with care or pose danger to the environment. When leaving the client, put the side rails up and adjust the height of the bed to lower position.

    AREA: Basic Nursing Skills

30. Maintaining a safe environment is part of the functions of a CNA. When arranging a client's room, you should do all of the following EXCEPT

A.　administer medications as ordered on time.

B.　check signal cords.

C.　adjust the back and knee rests as directed.

D.　check lighting.

ANSWER: A. administer medications.

RATIONALE: Nursing assistants are never allowed to give medications. This is a registered nurse's responsibility that cannot be delegated to a CNA. Performing this is considered malpractice for the nursing assistant.

AREA; Basic Nursing Skills

31. Its is important to practice standard precautions when

A.　Providing oral hygiene

B.　Dressing a client

C.　Feeding a client

D.　Ambulating a client

ANSWER: A. Providing oral hygiene

RATIONALE: Proving oral hygiene directly exposes the nurse assistant to the mucosa and oral secretions of the client which could be contaminated and possible source of pathogens. The use of gloves is warranted in the possible exposure to body fluids.

AREA: Basic Nursing Skills

32. Mr. Harrington is scheduled for cleansing enema this morning. What position should a client be in to receive an enema ?

A.　Semi-Fowler's

B.　Lithotomy

C. Left Sim's

D. Prone

ANSWER: C. Left Sim's

RATIONALE: Placing the client in the left sim's position facilitates introduction of the enema solution to the colon. The proctosigmoid area is located in the left abdominal quadrant of a person.

AREA: Basic Nursing Skills

33. Rapid heart rate, rapid breathing, and dry mouth are examples of which of the following categories of signs and symptoms of stress:

A. Physical

B. Emotional

C. Cognitive

D. Affective

ANSWER: A. Physical

RATIONALE: Rapid heart rate, rapid breathing, and dry mouth are examples of physical signs and symptoms of stress. These are directly physically observed with observation on client.

AREA: Mental and Emotional Needs

34. Those methods of disease treatment or prevention that are outside conventional practices are called:

A. Castigo de Dios

B. Yin and Yang

C. Shaman

D. Folk medicine

ANSWER: D. Folk medicine

RATIONALE: The health practices that re unique to a particular group of individuals are sometimes referred to as "folk medicine". Folk medicine has come to mean those methods of disease prevention or treatment that are outside the mainstream of conventional practices. Folk medicine is often provided by laypeople rather than formally education and licensed individuals.

AREA: Spiritual and Cultural Needs

35. From the following, choose the phrase(s) that is/are true regarding the way in which an individual demonstrates pride in one's ethnicity

A.  Placing value on specific physical characteristics

B.  Giving one's children ethnic names

C.  Wearing special items of clothing

D.  All of the above are true statements

ANSWER: D. All of the above are true statements

RATIONALE: All of these options reflect putting value in one's ethnicity which include acceptance and taking pride in racial physical features, using ethnic names and language, use of cultural garments and the practice of the rest of customs and traditions.

AREA: Spiritual and Cultural Needs

36. When developing a therapeutic relationship, a desired outcome is:

A.  Developing a friendship

B.  Making the client comfortable

C.  Moving toward restoring health

D.  Learning to know oneself

ANSWER: C. Moving toward restoring health

RATIONALE: A therapeutic relationship with the client is a helping relationship centered or grounded on the client's needs. The desired outcome is helping the client achieve optimum level of health or wellness.

AREA: Communication

37. An example of verbal communication is:

    A.  Moaning

    B.  Laughing

    C.  Writing

    D.  Crying

    ANSWER: C. Writing

    RATIONALE: Verbal communication is communication that uses words. It includes speaking, reading, and writing.

    AREA: Communication

38. An example of nonverbal communication is:

    A.  Speaking

    B.  Moaning

    C.  Reading

    D.  Writing

    ANSWER: B. Moaning

    RATIONALE: Nonverbal communication is the exchange of information without using words. It is what is not said. People communicate nonverbally through facial expressions, posture, mode of dress, grooming, and movements. Crying, laughing, and moaning are also considered nonverbal communication because they do not use words.

    AREA: Communication

39. An obstacle to effective communication would be:

    A.  Using the principles of touch by giving the client a back rub

    B.  Accepting what the client says while being alert to what he or she is not saying

    C.  Asking the client if he or she feels lonely or sad

D.  Interrupting the client when he or she seems to be deep in thought

ANSWER: D. Interrupting the client when he or she seems to be deep in thought

RATIONALE: Common obstacle to effective communication is to ignore the importance of silence. Allowing the client in silence will help him or her organize his thoughts and reflect on responses.

AREA: Communication.

40. When the nurse assistant stops in during the evening, Mrs. D. states that she is very worried about her operation tomorrow. Of the following responses, which would be the most appropriate:

A.  "That is very understandable, Mrs. D., would you like to talk about your operation?"

B.  "Don' worry- everything is going to be okay."

C.  "That's just a routine operation that you are having. No need to worry about it."

D.  "You'll be okay- your doctor and our operating room staffs do these procedures every day."

ANSWER: A. "That is very understandable, Mrs. D., would you like to talk about your operation?"

RATIONALE: Allow the client to verbalize or express concerns and feelings. To promote effective communication, the nurse aide should avoid "pat" answers that offer false reassurance. These are often misinterpreted by clients as a lack of interest.

AREA: Communication

41. It is suggested that the nurse sit in a relaxed position at eye level with the client when communicating with him or her because:

A.  This indicates that the nurse is fully involved in what is being communicated

B.  If the client feels rushed, he or she may interpret this to be disinterest by the nurse

C.  Responses to stress are manifested through active listening on the part of the nurse

D.  People have less control over nonverbal communication than they do over verbal communication

ANSWER: A. This indicates that the nurse is fully involved in what is being communicated

RATIONALE: Giving attention to what clients say provides a stimulus for meaningful interaction. It is best to position oneself at the person's level and make frequent eye contact. It is important that the nurse avoid giving signals that indicate impatience, boredom, or the pretense of listening.

AREA: Communication

42. For the visual impaired client, it is easier to read:

A.   Large print in black ink on white paper

B.   Small print in black ink on white paper

C.   Large print in blue ink on off-white glossy paper

D.   Small print in blue ink on off-white glossy paper

ANSWER: A. Large print in black ink on white paper

RATIONALE: When preparing reading materials for the visually impaired, choose large-size print in black ink on white paper. Letters and words are more distinct when they are set in large print with a typestyle on white paper provides maximum contrast and makes the letters more legible. Glossy paper reflects light, causing glare that makes reading more difficult.

AREA: restorative Skills

43. For the hearing impaired client, the nurse can facilitate communication by:

A.   Talking louder, using simple words, and lowering voice pitch

B.   Sitting or standing beside the client's "bad" ear when talking

C.   Selecting words that do not begin with the letters F, S, or K

D.   Raising the voice pitch, talking softly, and repeating the words

ANSWER: C. Selecting words that do not begin with the letters F, S, or k.

RATIONALE: Hearing loss is generally in the higher-pitch ranges. Selects words that do not begin with F, S, or K. these letters are formed with high-pitched sounds and are, therefore, difficult for the hearing-impaired person to discriminate.

AREA: Communication

44. Entries on the client's record should be objective, accurate, and legible because:

A. The client records are used by all health personnel in the health agency

B. The client's record are the property of the health agency and must be kept neat

C. The client has a right to read his or her chart; therefore, it must be legible and accurate

D. The client records are admissible as evidence in courts of law

ANSWER: D. The client records are admissible as evidence in courts of law

RATIONALE: Client's records are admissible as evidence in courts of law in this country. They are the basis for proving or disproving allegation concerning a client's care. Therefore, it is essential that entries on the records be objectively, written, accurate, complete, and legible.

AREA: Legal and Ethical Behavior

45. Of the following individuals, which one is most likely to have a higher-than-average temperature?

A. The person experiencing apathy and depression

B. The person experiencing an average day

C. The person experiencing anxiety and nervousness

D. The person routinely working the night shift

ANSWER: C. The person experiencing anxiety and nervousness

RATIONALE: Persons having strong emotional experiences, such as fear and anxiety, are likely to have a higher-than-average temperature. Conversely, persons experiencing apathy and depression are likely to have lower-than-average body temperature.

AREA: Basic Nursing Skills

46. The condition in which a person is aware of his or her own heart contraction without having to feel the pulse is called:

A. Arrhythmia

B. Pulse rhythm

C. Dysrhythmia

D. Palpitation

ANSWER: D. Palpitation

RATIONALE: The term palpitation means that a person is aware of his or her own heart contraction without having to feel the pulse. The pulse rate is usually rapid when palpitations are noted.

AREA: Basic Nursing Skills

47. The total amount of water that most adults consume each day is:

A. 1200-1500 mL/day

B. 1500-2500 mL/day

C. 1000-2000 mL/day

D. 2000-3000 mL/day

ANSWER: A. 1200-1500 mL/day

RATIONALE: The total amount of water that adults consume each day is about 1200 to 1500 mL. An additional 700 to 1000 mL per day is extracted from the foods eaten. As a result of metabolism, about 200 to 400 mL per day is added to the total fluid intake to bring it to about 2100 to 2900 mL per day.

AREA: Activities of daily Living

48. The oral hygiene practice recommended to break up bacteria lodged between the teeth is:

A. Using dental floss between the teeth

B. Directing a jet spray between the teeth

C. Rinsing the mouth vigorously with a mouthwash

D. Using an electric toothbrush regularly

ANSWER: A. Using dental floss between the teeth

RATIONALE: Many bacteria in the mouth become lodged between the teeth. The toothbrush cannot reach these areas well. Therefore, flossing several times a day in commended. Flossing helps to break up groups of bacteria between the teeth.

AREA: Activities of Daily Living

49. The term partial bath refers to:

A. Washing the area around the client's genitals and rectum only

B. Washing in a manner to remove secretions and excretions from less-soiled to more-soiled areas

C. Washing areas of the body that are subject to the greatest soiling or odor

D. Washing all areas of the body at the sink in the client's room

ANSWER: C. Washing areas of the body that are subject to the greatest soiling or odor

RATIONALE: A partial bath consists of washing those areas of sources of body odor, such as the face, hands, and axillae. Partial bathing may be done at a sink or with a basin at the bedside.

Area: Basic Nursing Skills

50. The first measure the nurse assistant must carry out when a fire occurs is:

A. Notifying the switchboard using the proper code

B. Turning off the oxygen supply near the fire

C. Using the appropriate fire extinguisher

D. Evacuating the people from the room with the fire

ANSWER: D. Evacuating the people from the room with the fire

RATIONALE: When a fire occurs, the first measure the nurse should follow is to evacuate the people ion the room with the fire. Remembering the shortened version of the steps as RACE will help the nurse: Rescue the people first before A, giving the alarm; C, confining the fire; and E, extinguishing the fire.

AREA: Basic Nursing Skills

# PRACTICE EXAM 2

1. When an accident occurs, which of the following steps should be taken first:

    A.  Report the accident to the proper person promptly

    B.  Comfort and reassure the client who was involved

    C.  Check the condition of the involved client

    D.  Call for the assistant of other health personnel

2. When an accident occurs, which of the following steps should be taken last:

    A.  Reporting the accident to the proper authorities

    B.  Entering all of the information on an accident report

    C.  Notifying the physician that the client has had an accident

    D.  Comforting and reassuring the client involved

3. A nurse assistant is helping in the care of stable clients in the burn unit. A thermal burn is a skin injury caused by:

    A.  Heat

    B.  Lighting

    C.  Steam

    D.  Electricity

4. The most prevalent type of accident experienced by older adults is:

    A.  Poisoning

B. Falls

C. Burns

D. Asphyxiation

5. Which of the following acronyms incorporates the steps found in most fire plans:

A. NFPA

B. RACE

C. ABC

D. OBRA

6. Risks associated with the use of physical restraints include:

A. Constipation, incontinence, infection,

B. Falls, confusion, asphyxiation

C. Dementia, disorientation, disability

D. Visual impairment, hypotension, urinary urgency

7. To avoid legal liabilities and maintain safe practice, you have to be cognizant of the scope and boundaries of your practice. Which of the following activities can a CNA perform?

A. Reprimanding another CNA

B. Supervising other CNA's performance

C. Mentoring and training other CNAs

D. None of these

8. After a meeting, the nursing director of the long-term care facility where you are working assigned you to take charge of the nursing home for three days because of a family emergency. Which of the following is your most appropriate response to the responsibility being delegated to you?

A. Politely ask for the details of the task

B. Assure the director that you will do what you can

C.  Contact the owner of the facility for advice

D.  Refuse the assignment

9. Mr. Enya has difficulty getting out of bed to sit on a chair and to attend to his bathroom needs. When assisting a client in and out of bed, the nurse aide should always

A.  get another person to help.

B.  pull the client's feet out first, and then lift the back up.

C.  put shoes on the client because the patient may slip.

D.  employ body mechanic techniques.

10. It is important to reposition your client on bed during an eight-hour shift to prevent immobility-related complications. How often should he or she be turned?

A.  q2h

B.  q4h

C.  q1h

D.  q1d

11. Which of the following is the correct procedure for serving a meal to a resident who needs assistance in feeding?

A.  Bring the tray into the room when you are ready to feed the client.

B.  Serve the tray along with all the other trays, and then come back to feed the client.

C.  Bring the tray to the client last; feed after you have served all the other clients.

D.  Have the kitchen hold the tray for one hour.

12. When making a bed or checking the linens of the client, the bed linen should be free from unnecessary bulk and wrinkles. The most serious problem that wrinkles in the bed linens can cause is

A.  restlessness or discomfort.

B.  disturbed sleep pattern.

    C.  decubitus ulcers.

    D.  bleeding and shock.

13. Which of the following statements most accurately describes a characteristic of pain:

    A.  Pain is objective in nature

    B.  Responses to pain vary widely

    C.  Pain is always associated with bodily damage

    D.  Pain is not a demanding situation

14. The client's discomfort is most likely relieved by a placebo in which of the following situations:

    A.  When the discomfort is only mild

    B.  When the discomfort is imagined or anticipated

    C.  When the client is almost recovered

    D.  When the client has confidence in his or her caregivers

15. The best examples of the vehicle of infection transmission in the facility are:

    A.  Nose, throat, mouth, ear, eye

    B.  Hands, equipment, instruments

    C.  Humans and animals

    D.  Any break in the skin

16. The single most effective way to prevent nosocomial infection is to:

    A.  Isolate clients with infections

    B.  Wash all equipment with detergents

    C.  Cover the mouth and nose when coughing

    D.  Practice conscientious hand washing

17. Gloves are required as barriers in which of the following situations:

    A.   When direct contact with the source of microorganisms will occur

    B.   To replace the need for hand washing when client care is finished

    C.   When microorganisms present on the hands grow and multiply rapidly

    D.   When the nurse assistant does not want to have contact with the client

18. It is recommended that the feet be separated in the standing position in order to:

    A.   Distribute the body weight evenly

    B.   Provide a wide base of support

    C.   Prevent the strain of locked knees

    D.   Relieves stress on the arches of the feet

19. Which of the following best defines body mechanics:

    A.   The efficient use of the body as a machine

    B.   The ratio of lean mass to fat mass

    C.   The structures of the body used for support and movement

    D.   The potential to respond when stimulated to work

20. The primary reason for recommending the "use of the longest and strongest muscles to provide the energy needed for a task" is:

    A.   This technique overcomes slouching and uses muscles properly to prevent strain and injury toi the abdominal wall

    B.   This technique uses gravity and reduces the strain placed on a group of muscles

    C.   This technique will provide the greatest strength and potential for performing work

    D.   This technique will provide a base of support and enhance the balance of the body

21. One should push, pull, or roll objects whenever possible because:

    A.  This technique will reduce strain and injury on the muscles of the lower back

    B.  This technique reduces strain on a group of muscles by using the body weight as a lever

    C.  This technique uses gravity and reduces the strain placed on a group of muscles

    D.  This technique improves balance by keeping the weight of the object close to the center of gravity

22. The reason for keeping the work area as close to the body as possible is:

    A.  Stretching will cause poor balance as the line of gravity falls outside the body's base of support

    B.  Stretching will cause strain and injury to the muscles of the legs and arms

    C.  Stretching will cause the client to feel uncomfortable because the nurse's movements are "jerky"

    D.  Stretching will make the nurse uncomfortable and therefore possible harm the client

23. Exercise is best described as:

    A.  The movement that accompanies the activities of daily living

    B.  The increased capacity to perform work with greater ease

    C.  The movement intended to increase strength, stamina, and overall body tone

    D.  The amount of movement that is possible in the normal joints of the body

24. Of the following types of exercise, which is performed with the assistance of another person:

    A.  Passive exercise

    B.  Active exercise

    C.  Aerobic exercise

    D.  Isometric exercise

25. Aerobic exercise is an example of which of the following:

    A.  Isotonic exercise

   B.   Isometric exercise

   C.   Therapeutic exercise

   D.   Range-of-motion exercise

26. Which of the following best describes rang-of-motion exercise?

   A.   Therapeutic activity performed independently

   B.   Therapeutic activity performed against resistance

   C.   Permanent loss of ability to perform therapeutic activities

   D.   Therapeutic activity in which joints are moved

27. For optimum use, a cane must be adjusted to an appropriate height for the client as follows:

   A.   The handle should be parallel with the client's hip, allowing the elbow to extend

   B.   The handle should be parallel with the client's hip, allowing 30° of elbow flexion

   C.   The handle should allow the client to lean forward 15° with the elbow flexed 10°

   D.   The handle should allow the client to stand straight with the elbow flexed 15°

28. When a client is using a cane, he should:

   A.   Place the cane about 10 centimeters (4 inches) to the side of the foot and hold it on the involved side

   B.   Place the cane about 10 centimeters (4 inches) to the side of the foot and hold it on the uninvolved side

   C.   Place the cane about 5 centimeters (2.5 inches) to the side of the foot and hold it on the involved side

   D.   Place the cane about 5 centimeters (2.5 inches) to the side of the foot and hold it on the uninvolved side

29. In which of the following situations would the individual use the three-point gait for church walking?

   A.   The client must be able to bear some weight on each leg

    B.   Weight bearing is allowed on one leg and no weight or only limited weight on the other leg

    C.   Weight bearing must be permitted on both feet, but they may have weak or limited ability

    D.   One or both legs are involved, and the client usually has leg braces or a cast

30. Which of the following are appropriate for walking on stairs with a cane?

    A.   Use the cane rather than the stair rail

    B.   Keep your back straight

    C.   Take each step going up with the stronger leg first

    D.   Move the cane forward with the stronger extremity

31. When using a walker, clients are instructed to:

    A.   Stand within the walker

    B.   Advance the walker 10 to 12 inches

    C.   Always step with the stronger extremity

    D.   Flex their hips and knees when walking

32. Restorative care begins

    A.   a week after admission.

    B.   as soon as possible.

    C.   when the patient wants.

    D.   twice a week.

33. You are told to put a client in Fowler's position. Before changing the position of the client's bed, you should

    A.   open the window.

    B.   explain the procedure to the client.

    C.   check with the client's family.

    D.   remake the bed.

34. During hand washing, you accidentally touch the inside of the sink while rinsing the soap off. The next action is to

    A.   allow the water to run over the hands for an additional two minutes.

    B.   dry the hands and turn off the faucet with the paper towel.

    C.   repeat the procedure from the beginning.

    D.   double the time of performing the procedure

35. You are going on a job interview in a prospective health care facility. How should you prepare to dress?

    A.   Wear your best jeans and T-shirt.

    B.   Use a lot of perfume.

    C.   Wear simple professional decent clothing

    D.   Wear a lot of jewelry.

36. For residents who have stress incontinence, which of the following techniques is especially helpful to restore continence?

    A.   The Crede maneuver

    B.   The cutaneous triggering mechanism

    C.   Kegel exercises

    D.   Intermittent straight catheterization

37. Of the following, which effect would a diet high in fiber and roughage have on normal intestinal elimination?

    A.   The production of a smaller stool and the promotion of quicker passage

    B.   The production of a larger stool and the promotion of quicker passage

    C.   The production of a larger stool and the promotion of slower passage

    D.   The production of a smaller stool and the promotion of slower passage

38. Constipation is best described as:

    A. A condition in which the individual is unable to have a daily bowel movement

    B. A condition in which there is a daily bowel movement of a small amount

    C. A condition in which the stool becomes dry and hard and requires straining for elimination

    D. A condition in which the stool is moist and soft and requires a laxative for elimination

39. Of the following, which foods would be the best for a client who has had diarrhea:

    A. Applesauce, coffee, and lettuce

    B. Bananas, bran flakes, and orange juice

    C. Bananas, applesauce, and gelatin

    D. Fried chicken, tomatoes, and tea

40. The nurse assistant prepares to measure a client's blood pressure. What is the correct procedure for measuring blood pressure?

    A. Wrapping the cuff around the limb, with the uninflated bladder covering about one-fourth of the limb circumference

    B. Measuring the arm about 2" (5 cm) above the antecubital space

    C. Wrapping the cuff around the limb, with the uninflated bladder covering about three-quarters of the limb circumference

    D. Using a bladder that is 6" (15 cm) long.

41. During assessment, the nurse measures a client's respiratory rate at 32 breaths/minute with a regular rhythm. When documenting this pattern, the nurse assistant should consider which term?

    A. Eupnea

    B. Bradypnea

    C. Apnea

    D. Tachypnea

42. The nurse assistant measures a client's temperature at 102° F. What is the equivalent Centigrade temperature?

    A.  39° C

    B.  47° C

    C.  38.9° C

    D.  40.1° C

43. When palpating a client's body to detect warmth, the nurse aide should use which part of the hand?

    A.  Fingertips

    B.  Finger pads

    C.  Back (dorsal surface)

    D.  Ulnar surface

44. Policy and procedure dictate that hand washing is a requirement when caring for clients. Which statement about hand washing is true?

    A.  Frequent hand washing reduces transmission of pathogens from one client to another.

    B.  Wearing gloves is a substitute for hand washing.

    C.  Bar soap, which is generally available, should be used for hand washing.

    D.  Waterless products shouldn't be used in situations where running water is unavailable.

45. Which of the following clients would qualify for hospice care?

    A.  A client with late-stage acquired immunodeficiency syndrome (AIDS)

    B.  A client with left-sided paralysis resulting from a cerebrovascular accident (CVA)

    C.  A client who's undergoing treatment for heroin addiction

    D.  A client who had coronary artery bypass surgery 2 weeks before

46. When moving a wheelchair onto an elevator, you should stay

    A.  behind the chair, pulling it toward you.

    B.  behind the chair, pushing it away from you.

    C.  in front of the client to observe his or her condition.

    D.  to the side and hold the door open.

47. The Foley bag must be kept lower than the client's bladder so that

    A.  urine will not leak out, soiling the bed.

    B.  urine will not return to the bladder, causing infection.

    C.  the bag will be hidden and the client will not be embarrassed.

    D.  the client will be more comfortable in bed.

48. Which of the following factors would have the most influence on the outcome of a crisis situation?

    A.  Age

    B.  Previous coping skills

    C.  Self-esteem

    D.  Perception of the problem

49. A client exhibits signs of heightened anxiety. Which response by the nurse assistant is most likely to reduce the client's anxiety?

    A.  "Everything will be fine. Don't worry."

    B.  "Read this manual and then ask me any questions you may have."

    C.  "Why don't you listen to the radio?"

    D.  "Let's talk about what is bothering you."

50. A client asks to be discharged from the health care facility against medical advice (AMA). What should the nurse assistant do?

    A.   Prevent the client from leaving.

    B.   Notify the nurse and physician.

    C.   Have the client sign an AMA form.

    D.   Call a security guard to help detain the client.

# PRACTICE EXAM 2 ANSWERS AND RATIONALE

1. When an accident occurs, which of the following steps should be taken first:

    A.  Report the accident to the proper person promptly

    B.  Comfort and reassure the client who was involved

    C.  Check the condition of the involved client

    D.  Call for the assistant of other health personnel

    ANSWER: C. Check the condition of the involved client

    RATIONALE: When an accident does occur, check the client's condition immediately. Note his or her condition and be ready to describe and address it accurately.

    AREA: Basic Nursing Skill

2. When an accident occurs, which of the following steps should be taken last:

    A.  Reporting the accident to the proper authorities

    B.  Entering all of the information on an accident report

    C.  Notifying the physician that the client has had an accident

    D.  Comforting and reassuring the client involved

    ANSWER: B. Entering all of the information on an accident report

    RATIONALE: After the client has been properly cared for and the nurse and physician have been notified, prepare an incident or accident report. All information related to the accident report. All information related to the accident is entered on the form. It is signed by the person completing the form.

AREA: Basic Nursing Skill

3. A nurse assistant is helping in the care of stable clients in the burn unit. A thermal burn is a skin injury caused by:

    A.  Heat

    B.  Lighting

    C.  Steam

    D.  Electricity

    ANSWER: C. Steam

    RATIONALE: A thermal burn, which is the most common type of skin injury, is caused by flames, hot liquids, or stream. Burns may also result from contact with caustic chemicals, electric wires, or lightning.

    AREA: Basic Nursing Skill

4. The most prevalent type of accident experienced by older adults is:

    A.  Poisoning

    B.  Falls

    C.  Burns

    D.  Asphyxiation

    ANSWER: B. Falls

    RATIONALE: Falls, more than any other injury discussed thus far, are most prevalent accident experienced by older adults, and they have the most serious consequences for this age group.

    AREA: Restorative Skills

5. Which of the following acronyms incorporates the steps found in most fire plans:

    A.  NFPA

    B.  RACE

C.  ABC

D.  OBRA

ANSWER: B. RACE

RATIONALE: The National Fire Protection Association (NFPA) recommends using the acronym RACE, which stands for: R=rescue; A=alarm; confine (the fire); and E=extinguish, to identify the essential steps in for rescue. ABC stands for Airway, Breathing and Circulation. OBRA is the Omnibus Budget Reconciliation Act.

AREA: Basic Nursing Skills

6. Risks associated with the use of physical restraints include:

A.  Constipation, incontinence, infection,

B.  Falls, confusion, asphyxiation

C.  Dementia, disorientation, disability

D.  Visual impairment, hypotension, urinary urgency

ANSWER: A. Constipation, incontinence, infection

RATIONALE: Although physical restraints prevent falls, they create concomitant risks for constipation; incontinence; and infections such as pneumonia, pressure sores, and a progressive decline in the ability to perform activities of daily living.

AREA: Clients Rights

7. To avoid legal liabilities and maintain safe practice, you have to be cognizant of the scope and boundaries of your practice. Which of the following activities can a CNA perform?

A.  Reprimanding another CNA

B.  Supervising other CNA's performance

C.  Mentoring and training other CNAs

D.  None of these

ANSWER: D. None of these

RATIONALE: The above activities belong to the roles and functions of the CNA's supervisor or the Registered Nurse. These tasks cannot also be delegated to CNAs by the nurse.

AREA: Legal and Ethical Behavior

8. After a meeting, the nursing director of the long-term care facility where you are working assigned you to take charge of the nursing home for three days because of a family emergency. Which of the following is your most appropriate response to the responsibility being delegated to you?

   A. Politely ask for the details of the task

   B. Assure the director that you will do what you can

   C. Contact the owner of the facility for advice

   D. Refuse the assignment

   ANSWER: D. Refuse the assignment

   RATIONALE: Taking charge of the facility in the place of the nursing director is over delegation and performance of the assignment is considered malpractice. As a nursing assistant, politely refuse the assignment stating it is not allowed in your practice and you do not have training for such task as a CNA, thus you don't have the needed competency for it.

   AREA: Legal and Ethical Behavior

9. Mr. Enya has difficulty getting out of bed to sit on a chair and to attend to his bathroom needs. When assisting a client in and out of bed, the nurse aide should always

   A. get another person to help.

   B. pull the client's feet out first, and then lift the back up.

   C. put shoes on the client because the patient may slip.

   D. employ body mechanic techniques.

   ANSWER: D. employ body mechanic techniques.

   RATIONALE: Body mechanics is the utilization of correct muscles to complete a task safely and efficiently, without undue strain on any muscle or joint.. You should always use good body mechanics when moving patients. Proper body mechanics are vital for prevention of injury and disability. Poor body mechanics are a major contributor to preventable low back injuries. Some of the most common injuries sustained by members of the health care team are severe musculoskeletal strains. Many injuries can be avoided by the conscious use of proper body mechanics when performing physical labor.

AREA: Basic Nursing Skills

10. It is important to reposition your client on bed during an eight-hour shift to prevent immobility-related complications. How often should he or she be turned?

A.  q2h

B.  q4h

C.  q1h

D.  q1d

ANSWER: A. q2h

RATIONALE: Turning or repositioning the client on bed every two hours helps prevent the development of pressure ulcers and thrombus formation. It can also help promote circulation.

AREA: Basic Nursing Skills

11. Which of the following is the correct procedure for serving a meal to a resident who needs assistance in feeding?

A.  Bring the tray into the room when you are ready to feed the client.

B.  Serve the tray along with all the other trays, and then come back to feed the client.

C.  Bring the tray to the client last; feed after you have served all the other clients.

D.  Have the kitchen hold the tray for one hour.

ANSWER: A. Bring the tray into the room when you are ready to feed the client.

RATIONALE: You should not bring the tray into the room until you have time to feed.

AREA: Basic Nursing Skills

12. When making a bed or checking the linens of the client, the bed linen should be free from unnecessary bulk and wrinkles. The most serious problem that wrinkles in the bed linens can cause is

    A.  restlessness or discomfort.

    B.  disturbed sleep pattern.

    C.  decubitus ulcers.

    D.  bleeding and shock.

    ANSWER: C. decubitus ulcers

    RATIONALE: The most serious problem that wrinkles in the bedclothes can cause patients is decubitus ulcers, or decubiti. The presence of unnecessary bulks or uneven linen surface with wrinkles add up to friction or shearing against the skin and can impair circulation underneath the skin and on the skin surface leading to pressure ulcers.

    AREA: Basic Nursing Skills

13. Which of the following statements most accurately describes a characteristic of pain:

    A.  Pain is objective in nature

    B.  Responses to pain vary widely

    C.  Pain is always associated with bodily damage

    D.  Pain is not a demanding situation

    ANSWER: B. Responses to pain vary widely

    RATIONALE: Pain perception occurs when the pain threshold is reached. Passing the pain threshold results in awareness of discomfort. Pain threshold tend to be the same among healthy people, but individuals tolerate pain differently. Pain tolerance is influenced by learned behaviors specific to gender, age, and culture.

    AREA: Restorative Skills

14. The client's discomfort is most likely relieved by a placebo in which of the following situations:

    A.  When the discomfort is only mild

B. When the discomfort is imagined or anticipated

C. When the client is almost recovered

D. When the client has confidence in his or her caregivers

ANSWER: D. When the client has confidence in his or her caregivers

RATIONALE: A placebo is an inactive substance given as a substitute for drug therapy. Studies have shown that placebos can be effective pain relievers when not used on a continuous basis and when the client has confidence in his health caretakers. It is wrong to assume that a client who as pain relief with placebos is a malingerer or is imagining his or her pain.

AREA: Restorative Skills

15. The best examples of the vehicle of infection transmission in the facility are:

A. Nose, throat, mouth, ear, eye

B. Hands, equipment, instruments

C. Humans and animals

D. Any break in the skin

ANSWER: B. Hands, equipment, instruments

RATIONALE: The vehicle of transmission is the mean by which organisms are carried about. Examples include hands, equipment (e.g. bedpan), instruments, china and silverware, linen, and droplets.

AREA: Basic Nursing Skills

16. The single most effective way to prevent nosocomial infection is to:

A. Isolate clients with infections

B. Wash all equipment with detergents

C. Cover the mouth and nose when coughing

D. Practice conscientious hand washing

ANSWER: D. Practice conscientious hand washing

RATIONALE: Hand washing is the most frequent used medical aseptic practice in health care agencies. It is the most effective way to prevent nosocomial infections.

AREA: Basic Nursing Skills

17. Gloves are required as barriers in which of the following situations:

   A.  When direct contact with the source of microorganisms will occur

   B.  To replace the need for hand washing when client care is finished

   C.  When microorganisms present on the hands grow and multiply rapidly

   D.  When the nurse assistant does not want to have contact with the client

   ANSWER: A. When direct contact with the source of microorganisms will occur

   RATIONALE: Gloves are required when an infectious disease is transmissible by direct contact or contact with blood or body substances.

   AREA: Basic Nursing Skills

18. It is recommended that the feet be separated in the standing position in order to:

   A.  Distribute the body weight evenly

   B.  Provide a wide base of support

   C.  Prevent the strain of locked knees

   D.  Relieves stress on the arches of the feet

   ANSWER: B. Provide a wide base of support

   RATIONALE: Keep the feet parallel and about 10 to 20 cm (4 to 8 inches) apart when in a standing position to give the body a wide base of support. One of the principles of body mechanics is to Maintain a Wide Base of Support. This will provide you with maximum stability while lifting. To do this: (1) Keep your feet apart; (2) Place one foot slightly ahead of the other; (3) Flex your knees to absorb jolts; and (4) Turn with your feet.

   AREA: Basic Nursing Skills

19. Which of the following best defines body mechanics:

A. The efficient use of the body as a machine

B. The ratio of lean mass to fat mass

C. The structures of the body used for support and movement

D. The potential to respond when stimulated to work

ANSWER: A. The efficient use of the body as a machine

RATIONALE: Body mechanics is the efficient use of the body as a machine. Using good body mechanics is as important for the nurse as it is for other. Basic principles of body mechanics can be applied regardless of the worker or the task.

AREA: Basic Nursing Skills

20. The primary reason for recommending the "use of the longest and strongest muscles to provide the energy needed for a task" is:

A. This technique overcomes slouching and uses muscles properly to prevent strain and injury toi the abdominal wall

B. This technique uses gravity and reduces the strain placed on a group of muscles

C. This technique will provide the greatest strength and potential for performing work

D. This technique will provide a base of support and enhance the balance of the body

ANSWER: C. This technique will provide the greatest strength and potential for performing work

RATIONALE: Use the longest and strongest muscles to provide the energy needed for a task. It is best to use the long and strong muscles in the arms, legs, and hips whenever possible. Small and weaker muscles will strain and injure quickly of forced to work beyond their ability. One of the most common injuries affects the muscles in the lower part of the back. It is a painful injury and usually slow to heal, but it is preventable when proper body mechanics are used.

AREA: Basic Nursing Skills

21. One should push, pull, or roll objects whenever possible because:

A. This technique will reduce strain and injury on the muscles of the lower back

B.  This technique reduces strain on a group of muscles by using the body weight as a lever

C.  This technique uses gravity and reduces the strain placed on a group of muscles

D.  This technique improves balance by keeping the weight of the object close to the center of gravity

ANSWER: B. This technique reduces strain on a group of muscles by using the body weight as a lever

RATIONALE: Push, pull, or roll objects whenever possible, rather than lift them. It takes more effort to lift something against the force gravity. Use body weight as a lever to assist with pushing or pulling an object. This reduces the strain placed on a group of muscles.

AREA: Basic Nursing Skills

22. The reason for keeping the work area as close to the body as possible is:

A.  Stretching will cause poor balance as the line of gravity falls outside the body's base of support

B.  Stretching will cause strain and injury to the muscles of the legs and arms

C.  Stretching will cause the client to feel uncomfortable because the nurse's movements are "jerky"

D.  Stretching will make the nurse uncomfortable and therefore possible harm the client

ANSWER: A. Stretching will cause poor balance as the line of gravity falls outside the body's base of support

RATIONALE: Stretching and twisting will fatigue muscles quickly. When stretching or twisting, balance will be poor as the line of gravity falls outside the base of support.

AREA: Basic Nursing Skills

23. Exercise is best described as:

A.  The movement that accompanies the activities of daily living

B.  The increased capacity to perform work with greater ease

C.  The movement intended to increase strength, stamina, and overall body tone

D.  The amount of movement that is possible in the normal joints of the body

ANSWER: C. The movement intended to increase strength, stamina, and overall body tone

RATIONALE: Exercise is the movement intended to increase strength, stamina, and overall body tone.

AREA: Restorative Skills

24. Of the following types of exercise, which is performed with the assistance of another person:

A. Passive exercise

B. Active exercise

C. Aerobic exercise

D. Isometric exercise

ANSWER: A. Passive exercise

RATIONALE: The preferred type of exercise is active exercise. People who are ill may need the assistance of another to move. This type of exercise is known as passive exercise.

AREA: Restorative Skills

25. Aerobic exercise is an example of which of the following:

A. Isotonic exercise

B. Isometric exercise

C. Therapeutic exercise

D. Range-of-motion exercise

ANSWER: A. Isotonic exercise

RATIONALE: Isotonic exercise is that which involves movement and work. One of the best examples is aerobic exercise. Aerobic exercise involves rhythmically moving all parts of the body at a moderate to slow speed without impeding that ability to breathe.

AREA: Restorative Skills

26. Which of the following best describes rang-of-motion exercise?

A. Therapeutic activity performed independently

B. Therapeutic activity performed against resistance

C. Permanent loss of ability to perform therapeutic activities

D. Therapeutic activity in which joints are moved

ANSWER: D. Therapeutic activity in which joints are moved

RATIONALE: Range-of-motion exercises describe therapeutic activity in which joints are moved in the positions that the joints normally permit.

AREA: Activities of Daily Living

27. For optimum use, a cane must be adjusted to an appropriate height for the client as follows:

A. The handle should be parallel with the client's hip, allowing the elbow to extend

B. The handle should be parallel with the client's hip, allowing 30° of elbow flexion

C. The handle should allow the client to lean forward 15° with the elbow flexed 10°

D. The handle should allow the client to stand straight with the elbow flexed 15°

ANSWER: The handle should be parallel with the client's hip, allowing 30° of elbow flexion

RATIONALE: For optimum use, a cane must be adjusted to an appropriate height for the client. When fitted correctly, the cane's handle is parallel with the client's hip, which should provide approximately a 300 angle of elbow flexion.

AREA: Restorative Skills

28. When a client is using a cane, he should:

A. Place the cane about 10 centimeters (4 inches) to the side of the foot and hold it on the involved side

B. Place the cane about 10 centimeters (4 inches) to the side of the foot and hold it on the uninvolved side

C. Place the cane about 5 centimeters (2.5 inches) to the side of the foot and hold it on the involved side

D. Place the cane about 5 centimeters (2.5 inches) to the side of the foot and hold it on the uninvolved side

ANSWER: B. Place the cane about 10 centimeters (4 inches) to the side of the foot and hold it on the uninvolved side

RATIONALE: The cane should be placed about 10 cm (4 inches) to the side if the foot. It should be held in the hand on the uninvolved side.

AREA: Restorative Skills

29. In which of the following situations would the individual use the three-point gait for church walking?

A. The client must be able to bear some weight on each leg

B. Weight bearing is allowed on one leg and no weight or only limited weight on the other leg

C. Weight bearing must be permitted on both feet, but they may have weak or limited ability

D. One or both legs are involved, and the client usually has leg braces or a cast

ANSWER: B. Weight bearing is allowed on one leg and no weight or only limited weight on the other leg

RATIONALE: The individual should use the three-point gait for crutch walking when weight bearing is allowed on one leg. The other foot cannot bear weight or can only bear limited weight.

AREA: Restorative Skills

30. Which of the following are appropriate for walking on stairs with a cane?

A. Use the cane rather than the stair rail

B. Keep your back straight

C. Take each step going up with the stronger leg first

D. Move the cane forward with the stronger extremity

ANSWER: C. Take each step going up with the stronger leg first

RATIONALE: When using a cane on stairs, use the stair rail rather than the cane to go up or down. Take each step up with the stronger leg, followed by the weaker one. Reverse the pattern for descending the stairs. If there is no stair rail, advance the cane just before rising or descending with the weaker leg.

AREA: Restorative Skills

31. When using a walker, clients are instructed to:

A.  Stand within the walker

B.  Advance the walker 10 to 12 inches

C.  Always step with the stronger extremity

D.  Flex their hips and knees when walking

ANSWER: A. Stand within the walker

RATIONALE: When using a walker, clients are instructed to stand within the walker.

AREA: restorative Skills

32. Restorative care begins

A.  a week after admission.

B.  as soon as possible.

C.  when the patient wants.

D.  twice a week.

ANSWER: B. as soon as possible

RATIONALE: Restorative care begins as soon as possible to prevent further complications. This is immediately started upon admission or consultation of the client.

AREA: Restorative Skills

33. You are told to put a client in Fowler's position. Before changing the position of the client's bed, you should

A.  open the window.

B.  explain the procedure to the client.

C.  check with the client's family.

D.  remake the bed.

ANSWER: B. explain the procedure to the client

RATIONALE: in all care or procedures to be done, you should always first explain what will be done and what are expected. The client has the right to know and to give permission to the performance of the activity.

AREA: Basic Nursing Skills

34. During hand washing, you accidentally touch the inside of the sink while rinsing the soap off. The next action is to

A.  allow the water to run over the hands for an additional two minutes.

B.  dry the hands and turn off the faucet with the paper towel.

C.  repeat the procedure from the beginning.

D.  double the time of performing the procedure

ANSWER: C. repeat the procedure from the beginning

RATIONALE: You have contaminated your hands and must start over.

AREA: Basic Nursing Skills

35. You are going on a job interview in a prospective health care facility. How should you prepare to dress?

A.  Wear your best jeans and T-shirt.

B.  Use a lot of perfume.

C.  Wear simple professional decent clothing

D.  Wear a lot of jewelry.

ANSWER: C. Wear simple professional decent clothing

RATIONALE: Your appearance is reflects your personality. You should wear the proper attire for the interview like simple descent business attire. Be sure to carry yourself comfortably with your clothes.

AREA: Legal and Ethical Behavior

36. For residents who have stress incontinence, which of the following techniques is especially helpful to restore continence?

    A.  The Crede maneuver

    B.  The cutaneous triggering mechanism

    C.  Kegel exercises

    D.  Intermittent straight catheterization

    ANSWER: C. Kegel Exercises

    RATIONALE: Strengthening pelvic floor muscles in one method for controlling some types of incontinence. It is especially helpful for stress incontinence and may extend the time needed for control in urge incontinence. The pelvic floor muscle exercises, also called Kegel exercises, increase the tone of the pubbococcygeus muscles.

    AREA: Restorative Skills

37. Of the following, which effect would a diet high in fiber and roughage have on normal intestinal elimination?

    A.  The production of a smaller stool and the promotion of quicker passage

    B.  The production of a larger stool and the promotion of quicker passage

    C.  The production of a larger stool and the promotion of slower passage

    D.  The production of a smaller stool and the promotion of slower passage

    ANSWER: B. The production of a larger stool and the promotion of quicker passage

    RATIONALE: The volume of the stool is affected by the amount of food that is consumed. A diet high in fiber and roughage producer a larger stool and promotes quicker passage through the intestinal tract. A diet low in roughage produces a smaller tool and tends to increase the time in remains within the bowel.

    AREA: Activities of Daily Living

38. Constipation is best described as:

   A.  A condition in which the individual is unable to have a daily bowel movement

   B.  A condition in which there is a daily bowel movement of a small amount

   C.  A condition in which the stool becomes dry and hard and requires straining for elimination

   D.  A condition in which the stool is moist and soft and requires a laxative for elimination

   ANSWER: C. A condition in which the stool becomes dry and hard and requires straining for elimination

   RATIONALE: Constipation is a condition in which the stool becomes dry and hard and requires straining in order, to eliminate it. The frequency of stool passage is not always a factor. Some persons may be constipated and yet have a daily bowel movement.

   AREA: Activities of Daily Living

39. Of the following, which foods would be the best for a client who has had diarrhea:

   A.  Applesauce, coffee, and lettuce

   B.  Bananas, bran flakes, and orange juice

   C.  Bananas, applesauce, and gelatin

   D.  Fried chicken, tomatoes, and tea

   ANSWER: C. Bananas, applesauce, and gelatin

   RATIONALE: To help the client who has diarrhea, the nurse should temporarily limit the consumption of food. Provide clear liquids until the number of tools and the consistency improve and then follow with bananas, applesauce, and light foods. Avoid fried foods, highly seasoned foods, or foods high in roughage.

   AREA: Activities of Daily Living

40. The nurse assistant prepares to measure a client's blood pressure. What is the correct procedure for measuring blood pressure?

   A.  Wrapping the cuff around the limb, with the uninflated bladder covering about one-fourth of the limb circumference

B.  Measuring the arm about 2" (5 cm) above the antecubital space

C.  Wrapping the cuff around the limb, with the uninflated bladder covering about three-quarters of the limb circumference

D.  Using a bladder that is 6" (15 cm) long.

ANSWER: C. Wrapping the cuff around the limb, with the uninflated bladder covering about three-quarters of the limb circumference

RATIONALE: When measuring blood pressure, the nurse should wrap the cuff around the client's arm or leg with the bladder uninflated; the bladder should cover approximately three-quarters (not one-fourth) of the limb circumference. Bladder size is chosen according to the size of the extremity.

AREA: Basic Nursing Skills

41. During assessment, the nurse measures a client's respiratory rate at 32 breaths/minute with a regular rhythm. When documenting this pattern, the nurse assistant should consider which term?

A.  Eupnea

B.  Bradypnea

C.  Apnea

D.  Tachypnea

ANSWER: D. Tachypnea

RATIONALE: A respiratory rate of 32 breaths/minute with a regular rhythm is faster than normal and should be documented as tachypnea. Eupnea is a respiratory rate of 12 to 20 breaths/minute with a regular rhythm. Bradypnea refers to a respiratory rate below 12 breaths/minute with a regular rhythm. Apnea refers to absence of breathing.

AREA: Basic Nursing Skills

42. The nurse assistant measures a client's temperature at 102° F. What is the equivalent Centigrade temperature?

A.  39° C

B.  47° C

C.  38.9° C

D.  40.1° C

ANSWER: C. 38.9° C

RATIONALE: To convert Fahrenheit degrees to Centigrade, use this formula:

$°C = (°F - 32) \div 1.8$

$°C = (102 - 32) \div 1.8$

$°C = 70 \div 1.8$

$°C = 38.9$

AREA: Basic Nursing Skills

43. When palpating a client's body to detect warmth, the nurse aide should use which part of the hand?

A.  Fingertips

B.  Finger pads

C.  Back (dorsal surface)

D.  Ulnar surface

ANSWER: C. Back (dorsal surface)

RATIONALE: To feel for warmth, the nurse should use the back, or dorsal surface, of the hand. The fingertips are best for distinguishing texture and shape; the finger pads, for assessing hair texture, grasping tissues, and feeling lymph node enlargement; and the ulnar surface, for feeling thrills and fremitus.

AREA: Basic Nursing Skills

44. Policy and procedure dictate that hand washing is a requirement when caring for clients. Which statement about hand washing is true?

A.  Frequent hand washing reduces transmission of pathogens from one client to another.

B.  Wearing gloves is a substitute for hand washing.

C.   Bar soap, which is generally available, should be used for hand washing.

D.   Waterless products shouldn't be used in situations where running water is unavailable.

ANSWER: A. Frequent hand washing reduces transmission of pathogens from one client to another

RATIONALE: Whether gloves are worn or not, hand washing is required before and after client contact because thorough hand washing reduces the risk of cross-contamination. Bar soap shouldn't be used because it's a potential carrier of bacteria. Soap dispensers are preferable but they must also be checked for bacteria. When water is unavailable, the nurse should wash using a liquid hand sanitizer.

AREA: Basic Nursing Skills

45. Which of the following clients would qualify for hospice care?

A.   A client with late-stage acquired immunodeficiency syndrome (AIDS)

B.   A client with left-sided paralysis resulting from a cerebrovascular accident (CVA)

C.   A client who's undergoing treatment for heroin addiction

D.   A client who had coronary artery bypass surgery 2 weeks before

ANSWER: A. A client with late-stage acquired immunodeficiency syndrome (AIDS)

RATIONALE: Hospices provide supportive, palliative care to terminally ill clients, such as those with late-stage AIDS, as well as their families. Hospice services wouldn't be appropriate for a client with left-sided paralysis resulting from a CVA, a client who's undergoing treatment for heroin addiction, or one who had coronary artery bypass surgery 2 weeks before because these health problems aren't necessarily terminal.

AREA: Member of the Health Care Team

46. When moving a wheelchair onto an elevator, you should stay

A.   behind the chair, pulling it toward you.

B.   behind the chair, pushing it away from you.

C.   in front of the client to observe his or her condition.

D. to the side and hold the door open.

ANSWER: A. behind the chair, pulling it toward you

RATIONALE: You must stay behind the chair to control it, but it should go on and come off an elevator backward to prevent the wheels from falling into the door opening.

AREA: Basic Nursing Skills

47. The Foley bag must be kept lower than the client's bladder so that

A. urine will not leak out, soiling the bed.

B. urine will not return to the bladder, causing infection.

C. the bag will be hidden and the client will not be embarrassed.

D. the client will be more comfortable in bed.

ANSWER: B. urine will not return to the bladder, causing infection

RATIONALE: Raising the bag above the bladder level can lead to backflow of the urine, with its bacteria, into the bladder.

AREA: Basic Nursing Skills

48. Which of the following factors would have the most influence on the outcome of a crisis situation?

A. Age

B. Previous coping skills

C. Self-esteem

D. Perception of the problem

ANSWER: B. Previous coping skill

RATIONALE: Coping is the process by which a person deals with problems using cognitive and noncognitive components. Cognitive responses come from learned skills; noncognitive responses are automatic and focus on relieving discomfort. Age could have either a positive or negative effect during crisis, depending on previous experiences. Previous coping skills are cognitive and include the thought and learning necessary to identify the source of stress in a crisis situation.

Therefore, option A is the best answer. Although sometimes useful, noncognitive measures, such as self-esteem, may prevent the person from learning more about the crisis as well as a better solution to the problem. The person involved could have correct or incorrect perception of the problem that could have either a positive or negative outcome.

AREA: Emotional and Mental Health Needs

49. A client exhibits signs of heightened anxiety. Which response by the nurse assistant is most likely to reduce the client's anxiety?

A. "Everything will be fine. Don't worry."

B. "Read this manual and then ask me any questions you may have."

C. "Why don't you listen to the radio?"

D. "Let's talk about what is bothering you."

ANSWER: D. "Let's talk about what is bothering you."

RATIONALE: Anxiety may result from feelings of helplessness, isolation, or insecurity. This response helps reduce anxiety by encouraging the client to express feelings. The nurse should be supportive and develop goals together with the client to give the client some control over an anxiety-inducing situation. Because the other options ignore the client's feelings and block communication, they wouldn't reduce anxiety.

AREA: Emotional and Mental Health Needs

50. A client asks to be discharged from the health care facility against medical advice (AMA). What should the nurse assistant do?

A. Prevent the client from leaving.

B. Notify the nurse and physician.

C. Have the client sign an AMA form.

D. Call a security guard to help detain the client.

ANSWER: B. Notify the nurse and physician

RATIONALE: If a client requests a discharge AMA, the nurse assistant should notify the nurse immediately. If the nurse and physician can't convince the client to stay, the physician will ask the client to sign an AMA form, which releases the facility from legal responsibility for any medical problems the client may experience after discharge. If the physician isn't available, the nurse should discuss the AMA form with the client and obtain the client's signature. A client who refuses to sign the form shouldn't be detained because this would violate the client's rights. After the client leaves, the nurse and nurse assistant should document the incident thoroughly and notify the physician that the client has left.

AREA: Clients Rights

Made in the USA
Las Vegas, NV
16 October 2023

79229720R00129